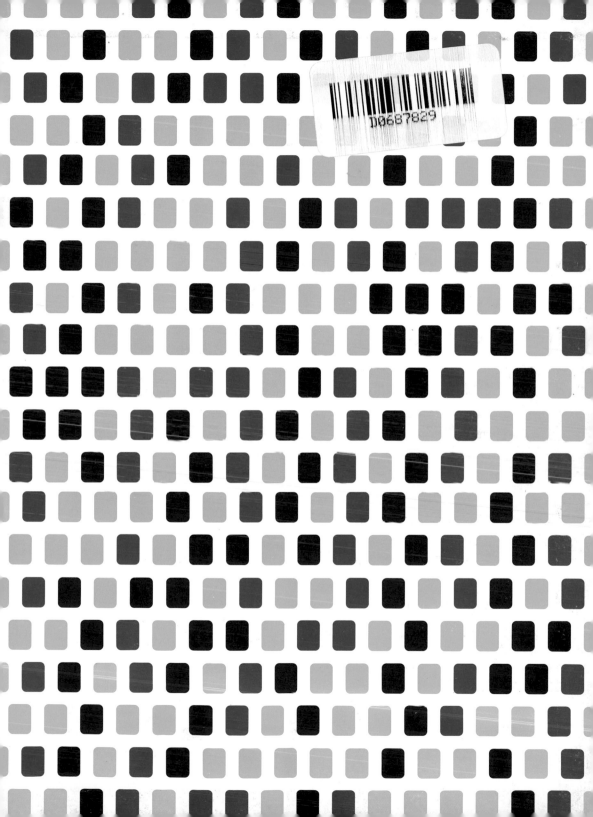

The Leafly Guide
to Cannabis

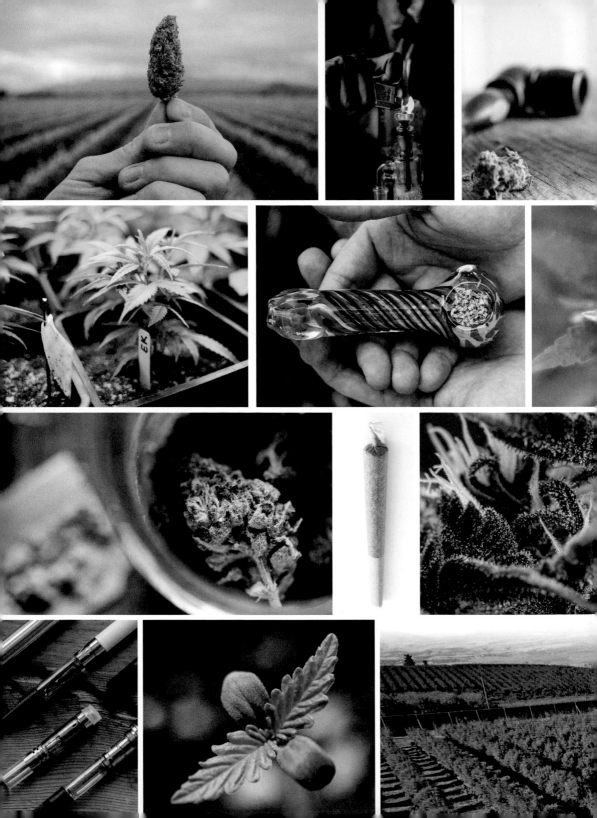

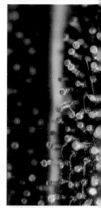

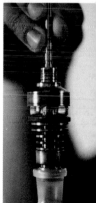

The Leafly Guide
to Cannabis

A Handbook for the Modern Consumer

The Leafly Team

TWELVE
New York   Boston

Twelve
Hachette Book Group
1290 Avenue of the Americas, New York, NY 10104
twelvebooks.com
twitter.com/twelvebooks

First Edition: December 2017

Twelve is an imprint of Grand Central Publishing. The Twelve name and logo are trademarks
of Hachette Book Group, Inc.

The publisher is not responsible for websites (or their content) that are not owned
by the publisher.

The Hachette Speakers Bureau provides a wide range of authors for speaking events.
To find out more, go to www.hachettespeakersbureau.com or call (866) 376-6591.

Library of Congress Cataloging-in-Publication Data
Names: Leafly.
Title: The Leafly guide to cannabis / The Leafly Team.
Description: First edition. | New York : Twelve, [2017] | Includes bibliographical references.
Identifiers: LCCN 2017029741| ISBN 9781455571994 (paper over board) | ISBN 9781478923572
(audio download) | ISBN 9781538711545 (ebook)
Subjects: LCSH: Marijuana–Therapeutic use. | Marijuana. | Cannabis.
Classification: LCC RM666.C266 L43 2017 | DDC 615.3/23648–dc23
LC record available at https://lccn.loc.gov/2017029741

ISBNs: 978-1-4555-7199-4 (hardcover), 978-1-5387-1154-5 (ebook),
978-1-4789-2357-2 (audiobook, downloadable)

Printed in the United States of America

WOR

10   9   8   7   6   5   4   3   2   1

For the advocates, connoisseurs,
newcomers, budtenders, and the
just plain curious.

Contents

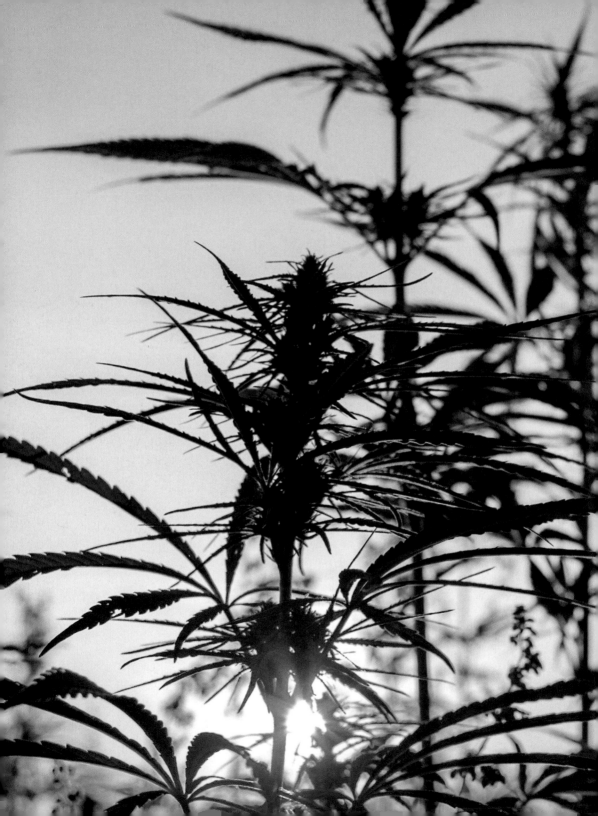

Introduction

Welcome to the New World

FOR MOST OF its history, cannabis has remained shrouded in code words, mystery, and misinformation. It's time we ended all that. This book, crafted by our staff of cannabis connoisseurs at Leafly, is your guide to clarity and understanding.

Cannabis, marijuana, weed, reefer, pot, ganja, joints, tokes, hash, blunts, dabs, wax, shatter: To those not steeped in the subculture, the jumble of terms can be as confusing as a foreign tongue. Relax. It's okay. That was their intended purpose. For decades, obfuscation has gone hand in hand with illegality. Before legalization, a cannabis sale required dexterity in a language as hidden as the space in which the transaction occurred. One did not simply offer up marijuana for sale, or request a half ounce of same. There were murmurs of "herb," "kine bud," "dime bags," and "Maui Wowie."

That strange argot served a double purpose. Vernacular fluency marked a buyer or seller as an experienced—and hence trusted—participant. It separated the authentic consumer from the undercover narc. In Richard Linklater's classic film *Dazed and Confused*, the endearing stoner Slater grills a newcomer to the scene: "You cool, man?"

Another character translates the Slaterism: "He was just asking if you get high." More to the point: He was asking if the newcomer could be trusted to not report the illicit goings-on.

The groovy terms also acted as brand names in a market that allowed no legitimate branding. When cannabis came in unmarked plastic bags, the seller's words were the buyer's only assurance of quality. Those words often conjured exotic locales—Panama Red, Acapulco Gold—that served to mask the poor quality of the Mexican brick weed under discussion. "Mexican brick weed" is a slang phrase for inferior cannabis, usually a mix of dried leaves, seeds, and stems. The name is taken from the way the product is pressed into brick form to be packed and smuggled from Mexico.

See? Now you know what Mexican brick weed is, and why to avoid it. Mystery solved. At Leafly, this is what we do.

• • •

Fortunately, for more and more Americans the days of plastic bags and brick weed are behind them. (Of course, you have to check if you're in a legal state first.) In most medically legal states, and in an increasing number of legal adult-use states, cannabis is grown by state-licensed farmers, bundled in smart packages, and sold in well-appointed dispensaries and retail boutiques. Cannabis flower—what you might have called weed—now appears in hundreds of varieties known as strains. An array of new products and delivery systems fight for space on the dispensary shelves: vape pens and oil cartridges, shatter, rosin, wax, edibles, inhalers, infused beverages, tinctures, capsules, suppositories, transdermal patches, and topical balms. Though regulations vary by state, most products are tested for potency and purity. All are backed by real brands, which means the market will reward the maker for delivering a consistent, high-quality product. Unlike, say, whoever stuffed that brick weed into the bag.

For experienced cannabis connoisseurs, the falling away of prohibition has provided long-sought relief from the constant fear of exposure and arrest. It's also offered an extraordinary side benefit: A vast expansion of product variety, enormous improvements in cannabis quality, and (surprise!) lower prices. Despite the imposition of exorbitant tax rates and an early spike in prices, improvements in efficiency have combined with good old capitalist competition to produce a legal market in which the world's finest cannabis is available at prices that undercut the illicit market.

For cannabis newcomers—or for those returning after years away—the new legal market offers both opportunity and risk. The opportunity lies in the possibility of finding just the right amount of relief, inspiration, or pleasure (or all three) for your body and mind. Past experience with cannabis of unknown origin may have soured you on the product. We hear you. We've been there. We also know that today's new products and exact dosages may click with you in ways that were impossible in the past. The risk? Consumption without knowledge and forethought can lead to sickness or at least a very uncomfortable night on the couch. In other words: Check the dosage before eating that cookie. Understand the difference between flower and concentrates.

How to Use This Book

The Leafly Guide to Cannabis is intended to help all consumers—expert or novice, medical or recreational—broaden their understanding and enjoyment of cannabis in all its forms. That said, more advanced consumers with years of experience under their belts may well wish to skip ahead through certain sections, such as How Does a Grinder Work? We encourage readers to make use of as many or as few sections of this book as they wish, depending on the information that is most pertinent to them. That said, it never hurts to brush up on the basics— you might find a fresh perspective on a familiar topic or pick up tips, tricks, and tidbits that you've never learned before! And remember, the use of this information may not be legal everywhere, so check the legality in your state before you use it.

Know your experience and your tolerance, and be fully informed before consuming. If you're seeking to treat a condition, be certain to consult your doctor before you make a decision.

• • •

We sometimes assume that everyone's post-prohibition journey begins with a first visit to a dispensary or retail store. But in most cases it actually starts with a conversation. It takes courage to break the stigma and discuss cannabis openly and without shame. But once you do, you'll discover that others are often happy to talk about it—relieved, even. And you'll probably end up sharing a laugh.

At Leafly, we aim to share accurate information about all aspects of cannabis. It doesn't happen just on the website: Friends, family members, and strangers who happen to hear of our work will ask us about medical marijuana, or topicals, or the new dispensary that just opened. We get asked questions in grocery stores, on airplanes, at football games, around campfires, and during Thanksgiving dinner. We're always happy to talk, because our own knowledge began with exactly these sorts of conversation years ago.

This book is our way of extending those conversations. We've gathered our best answers to the questions most often asked by the cannabis curious, along with many answers to questions nobody ever thought to ask (but wish they had). We invite you to use the following pages as a handy informational resource to dip into now and then or to read straight through. Share it with a friend. Share your knowledge with others. Expand all the good things: Curiosity, clarity, information, and understanding. Enjoy!

—*Bruce Barcott, deputy editor, Leafly*

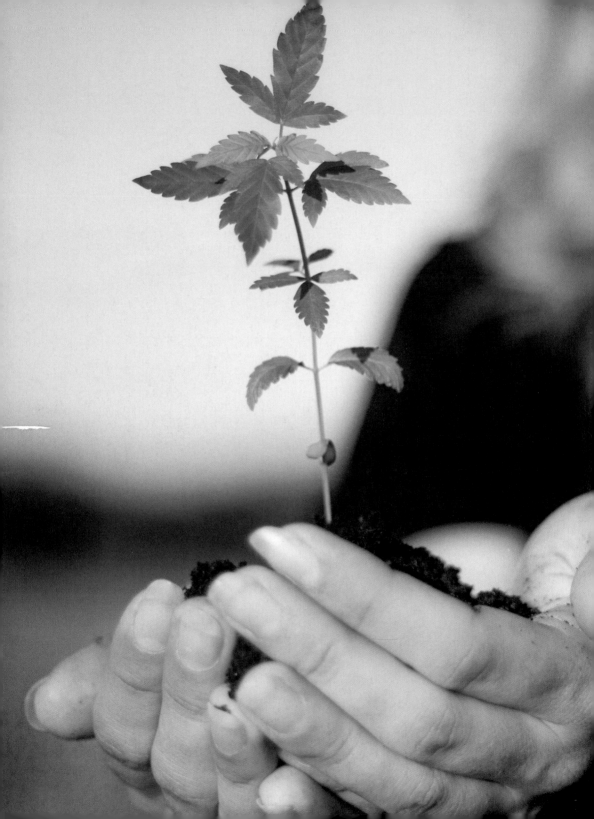

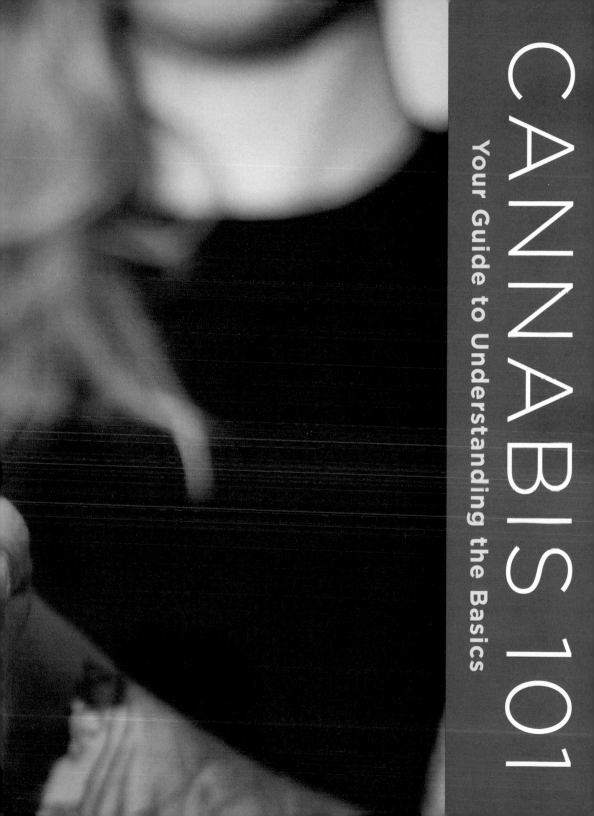

CANNABIS 101

Your Guide to Understanding the Basics

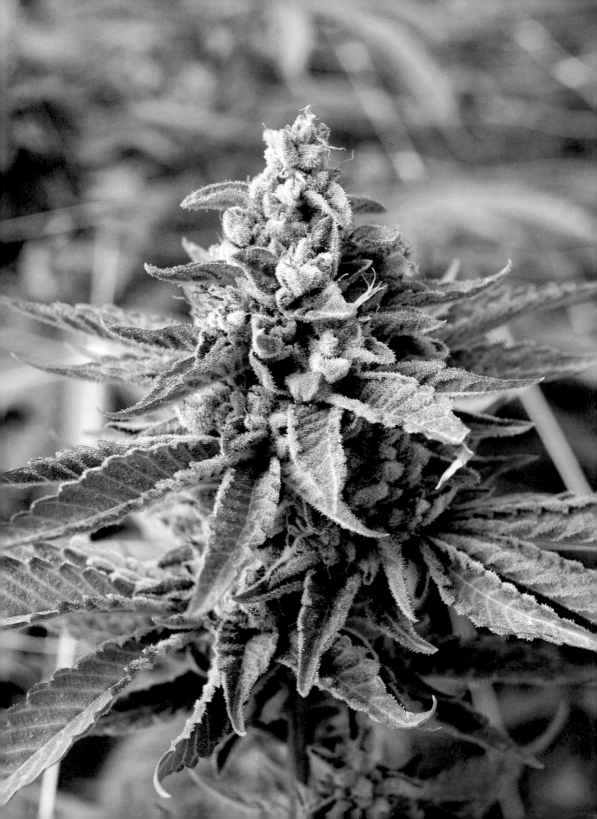

Sativa vs. Indica vs. Hybrid

What's the Difference Between Cannabis Types?

WHEN YOU WALK into a recreational cannabis store or medical dispensary for the first time, you'll notice a couple of things.

For starters, you've never seen this much cannabis in one place. And in so many different forms! Glass jars of bud, concentrate cartridges, tiny cylindrical containers of wax, colorfully packaged edibles, and tubes of topicals sit alongside glass pieces and smoking devices that run the gamut from discreet to disruptive. It's a cornucopia of delights for everyone from the novice to the expert.

The second thing you may notice is that the strains on the shelf are broken up into three distinct groups: indica, sativa, and hybrid.

Indica strains are known for being physically sedating, perfect for relaxing with a movie or as a nightcap before bed. Sativas typically provide more invigorating, uplifting cerebral effects that pair well with physical activity, social gatherings, and creative projects. Hybrids tend to fall somewhere in between the two, depending on the traits they inherit from their parent strains.

This classification has been around longer than you might think: early taxonomic distinctions between *Cannabis indica* and *Cannabis sativa* began in the eighteenth century when differences between their structure and resin production were first noted. The hybrid category was adopted as growers began mixing genetics from different geographic locations.

Indicas are believed to have originated in the Hindu Kush region near Afghanistan, where they developed thick coats of resin as protection against the harsh climate and conditions. Sativas thrive in temperate areas closer to the equator.

In addition to their different geographic origins, sativa and indica cannabis strains have several other unique attributes:

- Morphology—indica and sativa plants have different appearances.
- Flowering time—sativa plants have a longer maturation cycle than indica plants.
- Yields—indica strains tend to produce heavier yields than sativa strains.
- Flavor—indica and sativa strains tend to have different flavor profiles.

Two types of cannabis compounds—cannabinoids and terpenes—hold most of the influence when it comes to effects. Cannabinoids like THC (tetrahydrocannabinol) and CBD (cannabidiol) are molecular structures with their own unique properties and medical benefits. Terpenes are the aromatic oils secreted in cannabis resin that modulate the effects of cannabinoids, and these, too, have their own set of effects. In this way, cannabis strains are the sum of smaller parts, which may be passed on genetically. This helps explain the consistency in strain types, but there is still room for variation.

Let's take Blue Dream as an example. Due to its sativa-dominant genetics, we expect Blue Dream to make us feel uplifted and energized. Sometimes, however, you'll find a more indica-like phenotype, or a strain that expresses characteristics we associate with indicas, such as relaxing effects, a shorter flowering time, and a bushier plant structure. How the plant is grown can also affect the strain's terpene and cannabinoid contents, and more or less of either compound type may give rise to different physical sensations.

Our expectations must also be considered when it comes to perceived differences in strain type; when we consume an indica cannabis strain, we expect to feel calm and sedated, which plays into our experience.

As more research is conducted, our understanding of cannabis classification is bound to evolve as we learn what chemical configurations will produce these so-called sativa and indica effects. Until then, there's a wealth of user-submitted strain reviews to guide us to our next purchase.

Red, Purple, and Green: What Do Leafly Colors Mean?

You'll notice that strains listed in Leafly's database are categorized into three types and colors: sativas are red, indicas are purple, and hybrids are green. But does this mean that all red-tiled sativas and purple-tiled indicas are pure, 100 percent sativa or indica? No, not always.

While pure indica and sativa strains do exist, the market today is almost entirely dominated by a mix of the two, or hybrids. However, hybrids can be heavily sativa- or indica-dominant depending on their parent strains.

Let's take the sativa-dominant Super Silver Haze for example. This strain is not entirely sativa, given its indica genes from a Northern Lights parent. However, Super Silver Haze exhibits sativa-like attributes in appearance and effects, and is therefore considered a sativa-dominant hybrid. Strains showing a strong preference toward the indica or sativa side of the spectrum will be categorized as such on Leafly. Technically, almost every strain you'll ever encounter is a hybrid, but the red and purple colors on Leafly.com will help you determine which end of the spectrum that strain typically leans toward.

Cannabis Taxonomy

Where Do Indica and Sativa Classifications Come From?

CANNABIS SATIVA, C. INDICA, C. *ruderalis*—it's possible that you've already heard these terms used to describe different species of the cannabis plant.

"Cannabis" is an adaptation of an ancient word for the hemp plant and is the longstanding name of the genus that includes all hemp and drug varieties of the plant. "Sativa" is a Latin adjective meaning "cultivated," "indica" is Latin for "of India," and "ruderalis" is based on the Latin *rūdera*, the plural of a word meaning "rubble, lump, or rough piece of bronze." Ruderal plant varieties are those that pop up first in an area that has been cleared of other vegetation or barriers to propagation (growing "out of the rubble").

At first glance, these seem like fairly accurate descriptions for three distinct species. Humans have long cultivated what we consider to be sativa for its seed, fiber, and flowers. *Cannabis indica* may well have developed on the Indian subcontinent, and ruderalis is a feral, weedy

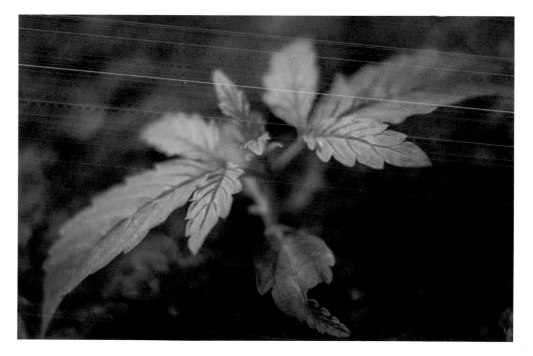

plant that thrives in harsh conditions. However, new discoveries and DNA analyses have provided a much more likely picture of how these species developed and how they are related.

To date, the history of the cannabis plant is still a bit of a mystery. The evidence suggests that it originated in Central Asia. Sometime near the end of the Pleistocene epoch, it migrated to small geographic pockets: one grouping in Western and Southern Asia, and one in what is now the Balkans and Caucasus Mountains. This represents the first major geographical split in the cannabis population, and is thought to be the main factor in producing two distinctly different species: plants bred and grown for oil seed and hemp fiber (Eastern Europe/Western Asia), and those selected for their psychoactive properties (South and East Asia). Geographical barriers like the Himalayan Mountains ostensibly kept these two populations separate for centuries, thus allowing natural and artificial selection to create two very different types of cannabis.

It's important to note that human selection is the most influential factor in the rise of these two different species. Ancient cultures in Eastern and Southern Asia had many available plants that provided fiber and food, so they selected cannabis plants for their psychoactive properties, probably as a spiritual aid. Conversely, western and northern cultures had fewer available sources of sustenance and cordage, so they selected cannabis plants for those properties.

Cannabis researchers are now starting

to coalesce around a system of taxonomy proposed by Robert C. Clarke and Mark D. Merlin in their exhaustively researched book *Cannabis: Evolution and Ethnobotany*. Using historical and recent publications as a launchpad, Clarke and Merlin produced the most thorough examination of the cannabis plant to date, using archaeological findings, historical accounts, and DNA sequencing along with their own personal findings and observations to present a compelling explanation for their proposed taxonomy.

The previously mentioned split between western hemp fiber cannabis and eastern drug cannabis proves to be the linchpin of this "rope versus dope" system. *Cannabis ruderalis* is considered to be either the ancestor of both of these types, or, more likely, a hybrid of this ancestor and some newer "escaped" cultivars. In their system, *Cannabis sativa* encompasses all narrow-leafleted, low-THC plants cultivated for hemp fiber and seeds, grown all across Europe and North America and in parts of South America as well. *Cannabis indica* refers to all varieties cultivated for their drug content, whether it's the broad-leafleted plants we associate with Afghanistan and the Hindu Kush mountains or the narrow-leafleted varieties cultivated in India, Southeast Asia, South America, Mexico, and Jamaica.

Decades of research by dedicated ethnobotanists and various methods of DNA analyses have helped to create what is probably the most accurate taxonomic structure to date. It may lead to a future change in vernacular used in the cannabis industry, but, for now, we'll continue

Indica vs. Sativa Effect Differences: Myth or Fact?

Nearly every cannabis store's menu is dividing into three categories: indica, sativa, and hybrid. They say that sativa strains are stimulating, indica strains are sedating, and hybrids can fall anywhere in between the two. But to what extent do these characterizations hold true beyond our own personal observations?

As commonplace as the three-pronged classification system has become, cannabis research—which is still politically suppressed despite the plant's growing legality—has yet to reveal a specific answer to us. Some researchers argue that the differences between the two are purely morphological—in other words, indica and sativa genetics have no bearing on perceived effects, only in their outward appearance. But some disagree, stating theories about possible chemical differences.

Terpenes, the aromatic compounds that give cannabis its various smells, may play a part. Secreted in the same glands that produce THC and CBD, pungent terpenes do more than repel predators and attract pollinators: they affect our experience. Individually, terpenes like myrcene and linalool are known to have relaxing qualities. Others, like pinene and limonene, are more uplifting. It could be that sativa strains produce more of these uplifting compounds while indicas offer more of the relaxing terpenes.

Cannabinoids, too, exert different effects. Cannabinol (CBN), a cannabinoid product of THC degradation, is known to have sedating attributes. THCV, another cannabinoid observed to have stimulating effects, has been found in sativa strains like Durban Poison.

The sativa-Indica dichotomy may be in part governed by terpene and cannabinoid profiles, but of course, personal physiology and expectations play a role as well. A new consumer trying a high-THC strain may have an entirely different experience from a seasoned veteran: They may find that strain to have sleep-inducing attributes whereas a high-tolerance consumer finds it increases creativity. Furthermore, anyone expecting an uplifting, energetic experience—based on how the product is packaged and advertised—will likely find themselves feeling stimulated.

It's likely that the perceived effects of strains have a lot to do with a combination of factors: chemical profiles, our expectations, and our unique biology. You may find that not all indicas sedate you and not all sativas energize you, but with enough trial and error, you'll learn to choose the strains you like beyond their indica and sativa stereotypes.

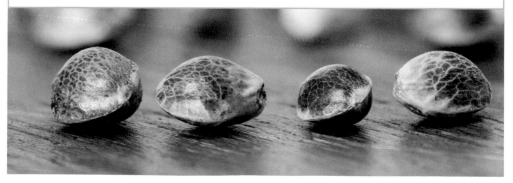

to refer to our bushy, broad-leafleted, sedating varieties as indicas, and our tall, narrow-leafleted, stimulating varieties as sativas. Using the new taxonomical nomenclature would surely present much confusion for retailers and consumers, so it's unlikely that the current meanings will be abandoned any time soon.

What Is Hemp and What Can It Do?

There are many different varieties of the cannabis plant. Hemp—also called industrial hemp—refers to the nonpsychoactive (less than 1 percent THC) varieties of *Cannabis sativa*. Both hemp and marijuana come from the same cannabis species, but are genetically distinct and are further distinguished by use, chemical makeup, and cultivation methods.

Hemp can be grown as a renewable source for raw materials that can be incorporated into thousands of products. Its seeds and flowers are used in health foods, organic body care, and other nutraceuticals. Hemp fibers and stalks are used in clothing, construction materials, paper, biofuel, plastic composites, and more. It's also more environmentally friendly than traditional crops as hemp requires much less water to grow—and no pesticides.

What hemp *can't* do is get you high. Because hemp varieties contain virtually zero THC, your body processes it faster than you can smoke it. Using hemp to put you on cloud nine will only put you in bed with a migraine!

Why Is Hemp Illegal?

In 1937, the Marihuana Tax Act strictly regulated the cultivation and sale of all cannabis varieties. The Controlled Substances Act of 1970 classified all forms of cannabis—including hemp—as Schedule I drugs, making it illegal to grow them in the United States (which is why we're forced to import hemp from other countries, as long as it contains scant levels of THC—0.3 percent is the regulation for hemp cultivation in the European Union and Canada). As a result of this long-term prohibition, most people have forgotten the industrial uses of the plant and continue to misidentify hemp with its cannabis cousin, marijuana.

The 2014 U.S. Farm Bill allows states that have passed their own industrial hemp legislation to grow industrial hemp for purposes of research and development. Several states—including Kentucky, Colorado, and Oregon—are already conducting hemp pilot projects. Many other states are currently pursuing similar legislation and programs. After many years of prohibition, American farmers are finally reacquainting themselves with industrial hemp.

In January 2015, the Industrial Hemp Farming Act (H.R. 525 and S. 134) was introduced in the House and Senate, where it remains at the writing of this book. If passed, it would remove all federal restrictions on the cultivation of industrial hemp, and remove its classification as a Schedule I controlled substance.

If the unwarranted federal prohibition of hemp is finally repealed, the world's oldest domesticated crop will once again be available to serve mankind in a broad range of environmentally friendly ways.

Cannabis Genotypes and Phenotypes

What Makes Every Strain Unique?

SOMETIMES YOU FIND a cannabis strain so good, you can't help but revisit the experience every time the opportunity presents itself. One day you might be surprised to discover a new batch of Blue Dream looks nothing like the one you last tried: what was once a spear-shaped flower now looks like a chunky bulb of crystal trichomes. It's the same strain, so what's with the variability?

Two things influence the structural formation of any given cannabis plant: genetics and environment. The plant's genetic makeup, also called a genotype, acts as a blueprint for growth: It allows a spectrum of physical possibilities, but it is up to the environment to induce these characteristics. The physical expression of a genotype is referred to as a phenotype, which is simply defined as the traits that the environment pulls out from the plant's genetic code. Everything from color, shape, and smell to resin production are affected by the environment.

This guide to cannabis genetics will carry you through the evolution of the cannabis plant, from its ancient beginnings to today's modern cultivation. By the end of it, you will understand that there are indeed defining characteristics for every strain, and each plant uniquely expresses its genes according to its garden environment.

The Earliest Cannabis Species

Cannabis is an ancient plant with roots all over the world. The earliest species are thought to have grown in the mountainous Hindu Kush region of Pakistan, while others later proliferated in tropical climates. These earliest varieties, called landrace strains, are considered the diamonds of cannabis genetics. Thousands of years of adaptation allowed them to express their very best traits in a very specific geographical location. These areas are what breeders like DJ Short call "sweet spots."

Our short, resin-heavy indicas populated latitudes between thirty to fifty degrees, whereas the tall, slow-growing sativas naturally grew in equatorial regions around thirty degrees latitude. These diverse habitats conditioned a colorful array of cannabis varieties, each with its own long-standing history.

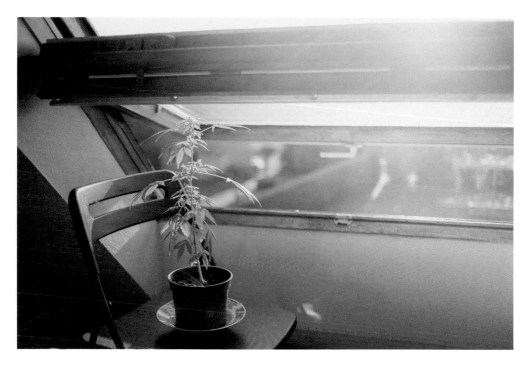

Cannabis Moves Indoors

Cannabis breeding took a major turn beginning in the 1970s and '80s when federal anti-cannabis sentiments peaked, driving cultivation from the great outdoors to underground. Indoor gardens, with raised soil beds, electric lights, and hydroponic systems, produce a bulk of the cannabis seen in the market today. While there's little doubt that masterfully grown strains have been cultivated indoors, experts will agree that the generic, unnatural environment can only bring out so much of the plant's potential.

Narrowing diversity even further, growers were primarily motivated by THC content and selectively chose this characteristic over other important chemical constituents like CBD.

In spite of this lost richness, we continued to see great variability in the plant's phenotypic expression: nutrients, temperature, the amount and angle of light, soil type, photoperiod length, time of harvest, and the distance between the plant and light source are among the many conditions that affect the plant's characteristics. Certain conditions may coax sativa- or indica-like traits, so as much as we love categorizing strains, we have to acknowledge that a strain's traits are not necessarily set in genetic stone.

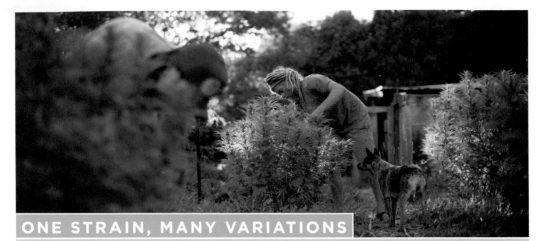

ONE STRAIN, MANY VARIATIONS

You'll notice that the same strain from two different growers may not look, smell, or feel quite the same. Why is that? There are several factors that can influence a cannabis strain from seed to final packaging:

Genetics: A plant's DNA plays a key role in the development of its effects, flavors, vigor, and growth attributes. Just like human and animal offspring, cannabis strains display a mix of traits from their parents. Stable genetics, achieved over generations of selective breeding, produce more predictable features passed down from the parent strains. If your strain's genetics are unstable, there is more variability in the outcome of the offspring.

Environment: Everything from the grow medium to the spectrum of light and its source, down to the pH and CO_2 levels, can change the outcome of your strain. What nutrients were used? Did the grower manipulate the plant's growth in any way? All of these are important variables that can affect the physical attributes of a strain.

Growing Techniques: The growing technique a grower selects also governs a strain's outcome. The same strain grown in soil, hydroponics, or aeroponics may demonstrate differences in the end product. A grower may also "train" their plants using techniques like low-stress training or defoliation. These manipulation techniques can change the final structure and potency of the plant.

Harvesting Method: The manner in which cannabis is handled during harvest time can completely sway the end result of your strain. Everything from the way the plants are flushed, when they are cut down, and even how they are dried can change the look and potency of each bud.

Curing: Curing is the process by which growers dry their crop after harvest, and this step can be the difference between good cannabis and truly exceptional buds. The curing process influences the outcome of the strain in a number of ways, most notably its flavor. A proper cure will break down the grassy flavors that are generally attributed to residual chlorophyll in fresh buds. Potency (the strain's THC or CBD content) and moisture content (more moisture creates a harsher smoke) are also affected by the curing process.

The Age of Hybridization

Hand in hand with the indoor grow revolution came hybridized strains, an intermixing of global indigenous varieties. This is when the sativa met the indica, beginning an ever-branching tree of hybrid offspring. Growers admired indicas for their resin-coated buds and short flowering periods, both of which are coveted traits for commercial production. The enjoyable, uplifting effects of sativa strains remain a genetic cornerstone, so mixing them with lower maintenance indicas seemed to bring out the best of both worlds.

If we think of indicas and sativas as falling on opposite ends of the genetic spectrum, it becomes possible to imagine the scope of phenotypic expression. Take Blue Dream, for example: A cross between the indica Blueberry and sativa Haze, Blue Dream may reflect characteristics anywhere on the spectrum between its parents, depending on how it was raised. This is why we sometimes see an indica-like phenotype of Blue Dream when we expect a sativa. That isn't to say strains are unpredictable genetic wildcards; rather, we just shouldn't be surprised when a strain does not fit perfectly within a categorical box. Again, it is possible to wheedle sativa or indica characteristics with specific conditions in a controlled garden.

Because of hybridization, we have a virtually limitless selection of strains to choose from, and avid strain collectors will always have new hybrids to chase. Connoisseur-focused growers may mourn the loss of original cannabis genetics, but many are still dedicated to their resurrection.

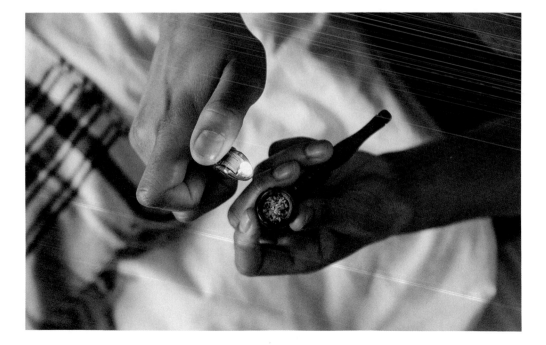

The Anatomy of the Cannabis Plant

WHEN EXAMINING A cannabis bud, you'll notice a complex knotting of different parts: the fiery orange hairs, the sugary crystals, chunky knobs enveloped by tiny leaves. But what exactly are these formations, and what functions do they serve?

This brief guide to cannabis anatomy is meant to familiarize you with the plant in its full form. Unfortunately, the sight of real, living cannabis is made rare by restrictive laws, so this guide should help bring you just a little closer to your favorite strain's source.

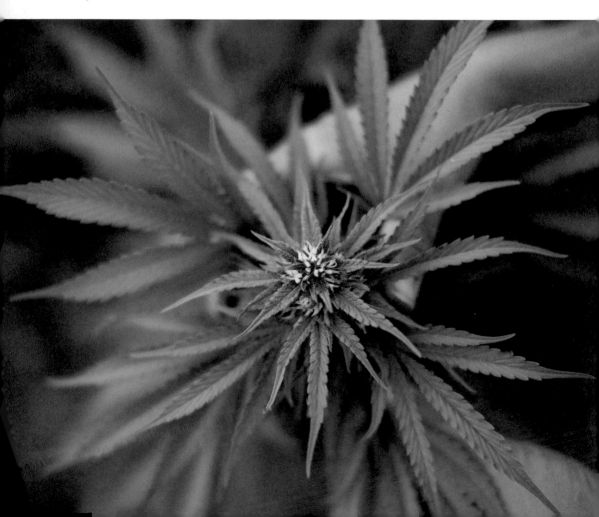

Males and Females

Cannabis plants can be male, female, or both (hermaphrodite), but what's in your stash jar are the flowers of a female plant.

Female plants produce the large resin-secreting flowers that are trimmed down to round or pointed buds while males produce smaller spheres near the base of the leaves. The male plants pollinate the females to initiate seed production, but the potent flowers we consume come from the seedless female plants, called sinsemilla, which grow large cannabinoid-rich buds without seed.

The rare hermaphroditic plants contain both female and male sex organs that allow the plant to pollinate itself during flowering. This self-pollination is typically deemed a nuisance among growers as it spoils the seedless sinsemilla plants and passes on hermaphroditic genes.

Growers can ensure the sex of their plants by growing clones or the genetically identical clippings from a parent strain. Feminized seeds are also made available through a special breeding process.

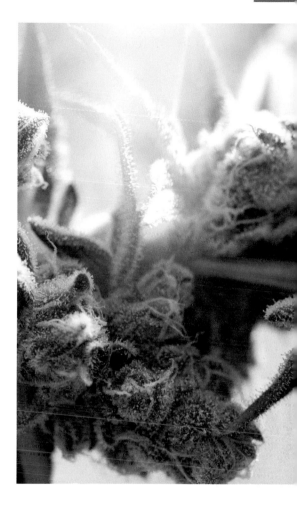

Seeds vs. Clones

A clone is a cutting taken from a plant and then placed in some sort of grow medium to induce root production. Once it has rooted, it can be grown into a mature plant that is genetically identical to the one it was cut from.

Seeds carry genetic information from two parent plants that can be expressed in numerous different combinations, some presenting more like the mother, some like the father, and many presenting various traits from both.

Generally, cannabis producers will plant many seeds and choose the best plant, and then take clones from that individual to grow their cannabis flowers, or simply start with a proven clone acquired from another grower as their mother plant.

The Parts of the Plant

The cannabis plant is comprised of several structures, many of which we can find on any ordinary flowering species. Cannabis grows on long skinny stems with its large iconic fan-shaped leaves extending out from areas called nodes. Cannabis really starts to stand out in the flowers where unique and intricate formations occur.

Cola

Also known as the terminal bud, cola refers to the plant's bud site where tight female flowers bloom. The main cola (sometimes called the apical bud) forms at the very top of the plant, while smaller colas occur along the budding sites below. The number and size of cannabis colas can be increased through a variety of growing techniques like topping or low stress training (LST).

Calyx

To the unknowing eye, cannabis buds just look like a knobby tangle of leaves, but the calyx is what actually comprises the female flower. Look closely underneath those tiny leaves (called sugar leaves) and you'll find a number of tear-shaped nodules. These are the calyxes, and they come in many different shapes, sizes, and colors. Calyxes typically contain high concentrations of trichomes, or glands that secrete THC and other cannabinoids.

Pistil

Out from the calyxes peek tiny red-orange hairs; these vibrant strands are called pistils, and they serve to collect pollen from males. Pistils begin with a white coloration and progressively darken to yellow, orange, red, and brown over the course of the plant's maturation. They play an important role in reproduction, but pistils bring very little to the flower's potency and taste.

TRICHOME

CALYX

PISTIL

COLA

Trichome

Despite their minute size, it's hard to miss the blanket of crystal resin on a cannabis bud. This resin (or kief when dried) is secreted through translucent, mushroom-shaped glands on the leaves, stems, and calyxes. Trichomes were originally developed to protect the plant against predators and the elements. These clear bulbous globes ooze aromatic oils called terpenes as well as therapeutic cannabinoids like THC and CBD. The basis of hash production depends on these trichomes and their potent sugarlike resin.

DID YOU KNOW? The purple, red, or blue hues seen in some cannabis buds are caused by pigment molecules called anthocyanins. Temperature and soil pH can change the color of cannabis flowers, but contrary to myth, color has nothing to do with a strain's potency.

What Are Cannabinoids and How Do They Affect You?

ONE HEFTY WORD that belongs in every consumer's vocabulary is "cannabinoid." Cannabinoids are the chemical compounds secreted by cannabis flowers that provide relief to an array of symptoms, both physical and mental. You might already be familiar with the two most common, THC and CBD, but cannabis contains over one hundred cannabinoids with different properties and uses.

Cannabinoids work their medicinal magic by imitating compounds our bodies naturally produce (endocannabinoids), which activate specific receptors in the brain and body to maintain internal stability and health. Simply put, they mediate communication between cells, and when there is a deficiency or problem with our endocannabinoid system, unpleasant symptoms and complications can occur.

When cannabis is consumed, cannabinoids bind to these receptors (called CB1 and CB2) throughout the body. Different cannabinoids have different effects depending on which receptors they bind to. For example, THC strongly binds to CB1 receptors in the brain, which is why we get a euphoric high. CBD doesn't

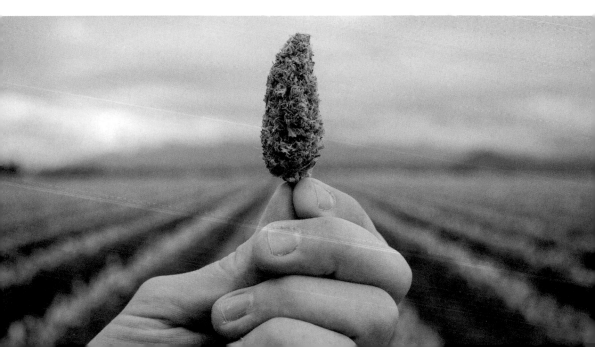

bind strongly to these receptors, hence its seemingly nonpsychoactive effects. However, just because it doesn't have an affinity for these specific receptors doesn't mean it isn't demonstrating immense therapeutic value in other ways.

The binding of cannabinoids to these receptors is the primary basis of cannabis as medicine, and is the reason cannabinoids can have so many positive effects.* The regulatory function the endocannabinoid system plays is exactly why some patients experience relief of pain, anxiety, seizures, nausea, insomnia, and so many other symptoms.

* You should consult your doctor before consuming.

The Endocannabinoid System

Cannabis works by binding to receptors throughout our body that affect various homeostatic functions—functions that help maintain internal health and stability. But cannabis isn't the only thing that binds to these receptors—naturally occurring chemicals such as anandamide and 2-arachidonoylglycerol (2AG) also bind to them. One example of these natural compounds at work is the "runner's high"—that's your brain releasing anandamide after a vigorous workout, and it can feel a bit like a mild cannabis high.

This system, called the endocannabinoid system (ECS), is a group of specialized fatty acid–based signaling chemicals ("keys"), their receptors ("locks"), and the metabolic enzymes that produce and break them down. These endocannabinoid chemical signals act on similar brain and immune cell receptors (CB1 and CB2) using the active compounds found in cannabis—cannabidiol (CBD), and Δ^9-tetrahydrocannabinol (THC).

We're beginning to see that a balanced and functional endocannabinoid system is essential to our health. When there's a problem or deficiency in our endocannabinoid system, the compounds in cannabis may help. This, right here, is the basis of cannabis as medicine.

What Is THC?

Most cannabis strains you'll come across are high in THC (Δ^9-tetrahydracannabinol). THC is the dominant psychoactive compound found in the plant, and it's the reason cannabis can make us feel euphoric, happy, and hungry. Too much THC can make for a bad experience, so always go slow and dose low if you're not certain how THC will affect you.

Today, most cannabis strains have a THC content of about 12 to 20 percent, but some of the more potent varieties clock in at nearly 30 percent. Some of you might be wondering why cannabis is so much more powerful than it was in decades past. In response to consumer demands for highly psychoactive varieties, cannabis breeders selected and bred plants that exhibited the most potency. Over generations, these heavy-hitters would come to dominate the gene pool, but as cannabis legalization invites new consumers, the demand for low-potency cannabis and high-CBD strains has also risen.

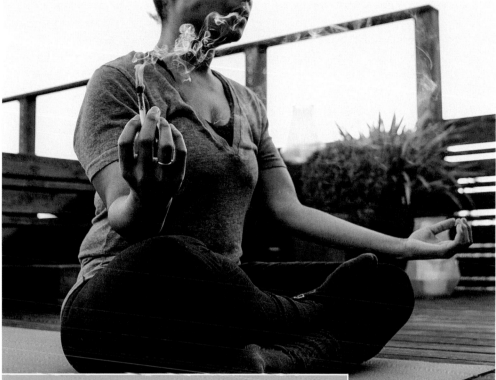

5 THINGS THAT ARE CHEMICALLY SIMILAR TO A CANNABIS HIGH

Catnip: Catnip is related to the cannabis plant, and like cannabis, catnip is thought to use its chemicals to confuse pests and predators. And no, humans cannot get high on catnip.

Running: Though commonly attributed to the release of endorphins, a "runner's high" is actually linked to the human endocannabinoid system. So not only is running healthy for you, it also mimics the high you get from your favorite strain.

Love: Scientists recently found that higher levels of oxytocin (a hormone associated with feelings of bonding) can release anandamide, an endocannabinoid that plays a role in the neural generation of motivation and pleasure, among other behaviors.

Chocolate: In 1996, researchers discovered that chocolate contains anandamide, as well as two substances that could mimic anandamide's effects, N-oleoylethanolamine and N-linoleoylethanolamine (yes, those are all actual words).

Cheese: Casein, a chemical found in cheese, can trigger your brain's opioid receptors and deliver feelings of euphoria similar to those delivered by cannabis.

What Is CBD?

CBD, or cannabidiol, is the second most abundant cannabinoid produced by cannabis. Delivering little to no psychoactive effects, CBD has risen in popularity among those who prefer a more mellow, clearheaded experience. You'll often find strains that have an equal amount of THC and CBD, a balance commonly chosen by those who are sensitive to the anxious side effects of THC as CBD itself exerts anti-anxiety effects. Any strain with more than about 4 percent CBD is considered by most to be a high-CBD strain, and varieties with only trace amounts of THC are often available in legal markets for anyone looking for relaxation without the high.

Adult recreational consumers aren't the only ones swarming toward high-CBD strains. Those in research and medicine are vigorously experimenting with CBD as a compound with immense pharmacological promise. Widely known for its anti-seizure properties in pediatric epilepsy, CBD may also be an effective treatment for anxiety, addiction, multiple sclerosis, pain, inflammation, and other conditions.

Some of the most popular CBD varieties to look out for include ACDC, Cannatonic, Harle-Tsu, Canna-Tsu, and Harlequin.

Other Cannabinoids at a Glance

CBN: A sedating, sleepy cannabinoid that is found in higher amounts in aged cannabis as THC degrades.

CBC: A nonpsychoactive cannabinoid being studied for its antianxiety and anti-inflammatory properties.

THCA: The nonpsychoactive precursor to THC found in raw cannabis, THCA is known to have anti-inflammatory, neuroprotective, and antinausea effects. Raw cannabis leaves are popularly juiced or brewed into teas for their THCA content.

THCV: Thought to have high-energy psychoactive effects, THCV is an appetite-suppressing, anxiety-fighting cannabinoid holding promise for conditions like diabetes, PTSD, Alzheimer's disease, and osteoporosis.

What Are Terpenes and How Do They Impact Cannabis Strains?

THERE'S SOMETHING ABOUT the aroma of cannabis that soothes the mind and body. Whether it's the sweet fruity taste of Pineapple Express or that skunky smell that bursts from a cracked bud of Sour Diesel, we know there's something going on under their complex and flavorful bouquets.

Terpenes are what you smell, and knowing what they are will deepen your appreciation of cannabis, regardless of whether you're a medical patient or a recreational consumer.

Secreted in the same glands that produce cannabinoids like THC and CBD, terpenes are the pungent oils that distinguish

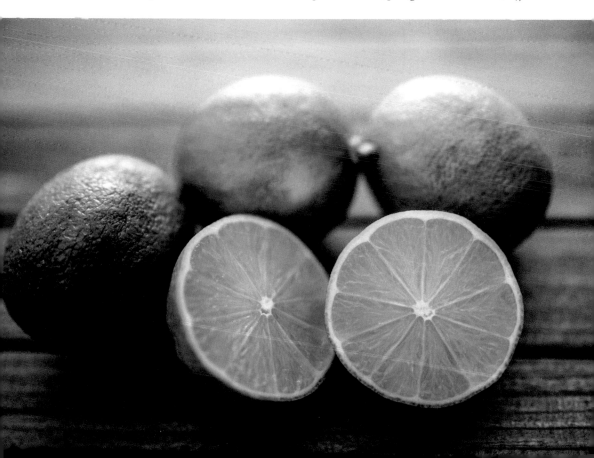

cannabis varieties with distinctive flavors like citrus, berry, mint, and pine.

Not unlike other strong-smelling plants and flowers, the development of terpenes in cannabis began for adaptive purposes: to repel predators and lure pollinators. There are many factors that influence a plant's development of terpenes, including climate, weather, age and maturation, fertilizers, and soil type.

More than a hundred different terpenes have been identified in the cannabis plant, and every strain tends toward a unique terpene type and composition. In other words, a strain like Cheese and its descendants will likely have a discernible cheeselike smell, and Blueberry offspring will often inherit the scent of berries.

The diverse palate of cannabis flavors is impressive enough, but arguably the most fascinating characteristic of terpenes is their ability to interact synergistically with other compounds in the plant, like cannabinoids. In the past few decades, most cannabis varieties have been bred to contain high levels of THC, and as a result, other cannabinoids like CBD have fallen to just trace amounts. This has led many to believe that terpenes may play

DID YOU KNOW? Terpenes are highly volatile, easily combustible compounds. To best preserve these tasty terpenes, consume cannabis with a vaporizer. Vaporizers heat cannabis at lower temperatures, so you get more THC, CBD, and terpenes without the smoke.

a key role in differentiating the effects of various cannabis strains.

THC binds to cannabinoid receptors concentrated heavily in the brain where psychoactive effects are produced. Some terpenes also bind to these receptor sites and affect their chemical output. Others can modify how much THC passes through the blood-brain barrier. Their hand of influence even reaches to neurotransmitters like dopamine and serotonin by altering their rate of production and destruction, their movement, and availability of receptors.

The effects these mechanisms produce vary from terpene to terpene; some are especially successful in relieving stress, while others promote focus and acuity. Myrcene, for example, induces sleep whereas limonene elevates mood. There are also effects that are imperceptible, like the gastro-protective properties of caryophyllene.

Their differences can be subtle, but terpenes add great depth to the horticultural art and connoisseurship of cannabis. Most importantly, terpenes may offer additional medical value as they mediate our body's interaction with therapeutic cannabinoids. Many cannabis analysis labs now test terpene content, so any consumer can have a better idea of what effects a strain might produce. With their unlimited combinations of synergistic effects, terpenes will likely open up new scientific and medical terrains for cannabis research.

Most Common Cannabis Terpenes

Pinene

Aroma: Pine

Common Effects: Alertness, memory retention, counteracts some THC effects

Potential Medical Value: Asthma relief, antiseptic, anti-inflammatory

Also Found In: Pine needles, rosemary, basil, parsley, dill

Cannabis Strains with a High Pinene Potential: Jack Herer, Chemdawg, Trainwreck, Super Silver Haze, White Widow, Island Sweet Skunk, Blue Dream

DID YOU KNOW? Pinene is the most commonly encountered terpene in nature.

Myrcene

Aroma: Musky, cloves, earthy, herbal with notes of citrus and tropical fruit

Common Effects: Sedating "couch-lock" effect, relaxing

Potential Medical Value: Antioxidant; relieves muscle tension, sleeplessness, pain, inflammation, and depression

Also Found In: Mango, lemongrass, thyme, hops

Cannabis Strains with a High Myrcene Potential: Granddaddy Purple, Banana Kush, ACDC, Purple Kush, White Fire OG, Space Queen, Skywalker OG, Grape Ape

FUN FACT Ever been told to eat a mango if you want to enhance your high? The logic here is that mangoes contain a high level of myrcene. Try it out next time you have a mango.

Limonene

Aroma: Citrus

Common Effects: Elevated mood, stress relief

Potential Medical Value: Antifungal; antibacterial; anticarcinogenic; mood enhancement; may treat gastrointestinal complications, heartburn, and depression

Also Found In: Fruit rinds, rosemary, juniper, peppermint

Cannabis Strains with a High Limonene Potential: Durban Poison, Golden Goat, Trainwreck, Super Lemon Haze, Sour Diesel, LA Confidential, Headband, Alien OG

Caryophyllene

Aroma: Pepper, spicy, woody, cloves

Common Effects: No detectable physical effects

Potential Medical Value: Gastro-protective, anti-inflammatory; good for arthritis, ulcers, autoimmune disorders, and gastrointestinal complications

Also Found In: Black pepper, cloves, cotton

Cannabis Strains with a High Caryophyllene Potential: Hash Plant, Tahoe OG Kush, Girl Scout Cookies, ACDC

Linalool

Aroma: Floral, citrus, candy

Common Effects: Anxiety relief and sedation

Potential Medical Value: Antianxiety, anticonvulsant, antidepressant, antiacne

Also Found In: Lavender, citrus, birch, laurel, rosewood

Cannabis Strains with a High Linalool Potential: G13, Amnesia Haze, Lavender, LA Confidential

▶ Terpenes at a Glance

	MYRCENE	CARYOPHYLLENE	LINALOOL	PINENE	HUMULENE	LIMONENE
BOILING POINTS	168°C (334°F)	168°C (320°F)	198°C (388°F)	155°C (311°F)	198°C (388°F)	176°C (349°F)
AROMAS	musk, cloves, herbal, citrus	pepper, wood, spice	floral, citrus, spice	sharp, sweet, pine	woody, earthy	citrus, lemon, orange
EFFECTS	sedating, relaxing, enhances THC's psychoactivity	no detectable physical effects	sedating, calming	memory retention, alertness	suppresses appetite	elevated mood, stress relief
ALSO FOUND IN	mango, thyme, citrus, lemongrass, bay leaves	pepper, cloves, hops, basil, oregano	lavender, citrus, laurel, birch, rosewood	pine needles, conifers, sage	hops, coriander	citrus rinds, juniper, peppermint
MEDICAL BENEFITS	antiseptic, anti-bacterial, antifungal, inflammation	antioxidant, inflammation, muscle spasms, pain, insomnia	insomnia stress, depression, anxiety, pain, convulsions	inflammation, asthma (bronchiodilator)	anti-inflamatory, anti-bacterial, pain	anti-depression, anti-anxiety, gastric reflux, antifungal

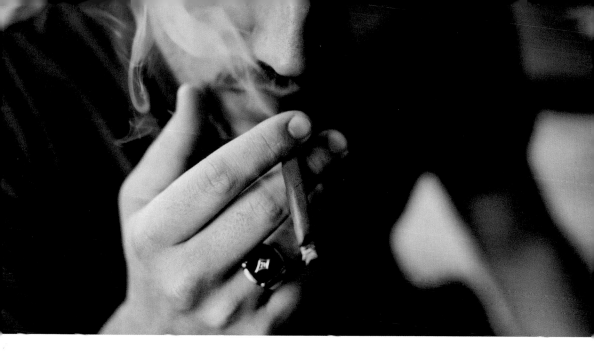

A Definitive Guide to Leafly's Top Strains

Once upon a time, cannabis was delivered to us, nameless, in a plastic bag. If your dealer bothered to provide a name, maybe it was called OG Kush, Blue Dream, or Northern Lights. Today, as we gaze upon walls stacked with legal cannabis, you'd be hard-pressed to find one that *didn't* have a name. So where did strain names come from, and what exactly do they mean?

While legal cannabis may be relatively new, the art and science of cannabis breeding is not. Decades ago, hushed grow operations were using strain names as a way to describe their personal creation. Some strains long separated from their original cultivators may have been given a name by whichever random consumer decided to give it one and share it. However a strain got its name, it received it for a single functional purpose: to differentiate it from other cannabis that was namelessly floating about the market.

Today, there are thousands of different named cannabis varieties—so many that a database like Leafly must exist in order to keep them straight! As an easy introduction to the world of cannabis strains, we decided to introduce you to our top twenty, with each one bringing something special to the table.

> **Editor's Note:** The best efforts were made to ensure the proper vetting of the origins of these strains. However, as we mentioned, cannabis history is pretty hazy. If anyone has more information on the origin of any of these or any other strains on Leafly, please don't hesitate to reach out to us—we'd love to talk. We have also noted the most common effects, but effects may vary widely, so consult your doctor (and check the legality of your location) before medicating.

Blue Dream

"Incredible strain, especially for wanting to get activities and responsibilities done. It provides a very energetic and alert high that will give you an adventurous demeanor."

The most common and illustrious strain found across the United States.

Parent Strains: Blueberry x Haze

Flavors: Mixed berries with pronounced blueberry notes

Description: Blue Dream, a sativa-dominant hybrid originating in California, has achieved legendary status across the United States. Crossing a Blueberry indica with the sativa Haze, Blue Dream balances full-body relaxation with gentle cerebral invigoration. Novice and veteran consumers alike enjoy the level effects of Blue Dream, which ease you gently into a calm euphoria. Some Blue Dream phenotypes express a more indica-like look and feel, but the sativa-leaning variety remains most prevalent.

Consumption Tips: New to cannabis? Blue Dream is a fantastic strain for those seeking a gentle, mellow high without the anxious edge. For an even more mellow psychoactive experience, mix this strain with a high-CBD variety.

Best Pairings: Blue Dream is a versatile strain that suits rainy, lazy days at home just as much as sunny mornings spent outdoors. Roll it up and bring it on a hike, or share it with friends at your next movie night. Use it as a dessert strain following a big dinner, or pair it with your favorite wine or beer to bring out the sweet berry notes.

Recommended Vaping Temperatures:

- 330°F for uplifting, creative effects
- 360°F for relaxed mind and body

OG Kush

"It tastes delicious almost like a woody vanilla with sort of sweet undertone . . . I was so happy and talkative when usually I'm sort of antisocial. This bud kept a smile on my face and kept me giggling."

The strain that gave rise to countless famous West Coast hybrids.

Parent Strains: Unknown

Flavors: Earthy pine with undertones of sour lemon zest

Description: OG Kush makes up the genetic backbone of West Coast cannabis varieties, but in spite of its ubiquity, its genetic origins remain a mystery. Popular myth maintains that Chemdawg and Hindu Kush parented OG Kush, passing on the distinct "kush" bud structure we see in many strains today. However, we can't be sure because OG Kush first came from bag seed in the early '90s. The earliest propagators (now known as Imperial Genetics) are said to have brought the seeds out of Florida to Colorado and Southern California, where it now flourishes. OG Kush is cherished for its ability to crush stress under the weight of its heavy euphoria.

Consumption Tips: Known for a pronounced THC content that often stretches beyond 20 percent, unseasoned consumers should tread carefully with this heavyweight. For those who can stand the potency, this one is a favorite for rolling into joints and blunts.

Best Pairings: Though small doses may still leave you feeling functional and active, OG Kush is best paired with relaxing activities. Spark it up in the hot tub or bath, or let it fuel your next movie binge.

Recommended Vaping Temperatures:

- 350°F for relaxed mood elevation
- 395°F for deeply sedating, heavily euphoric effects

Sativa

Sd

Sour Diesel

Sour Diesel

"Extremely cerebral whenever I consumed it, but, as many others have pointed out, there really is no 'couch-lock.' It's almost like Sour Diesel is a key, a key that opens up whole realms of your mind that you were once ignorant of."

A popular sativa-dominant hybrid that smells just like its name.

Parent Strains: Unknown

Flavors: Sour lemon meets pungent, gassy diesel

Description: Sour Diesel, nicknamed Sour D, is most popularly known as a sativa-leaning hybrid with invigorating effects that put a pep in your step. But although most Sour Diesels today are sativa-like in appearance and effect, the original Sour Diesel from New York is said to be a hybrid with balanced effects inherited from Chemdawg 91 and Super Skunk. With so many look-alikes circulating the market, tracing Sour Diesel's lineage has become somewhat of a murky endeavor. Most Sour Diesel you'll come across, however, will carry a distinct diesel aroma that gave this strain its name and will have light-footed effects that'll float you straight to cloud nine.

Consumption Tips: Love that Sour Diesel flavor? Put it in a vaporizer for the best flavor preservation. Despise that nasty fuel taste, but love Sour D's effects? Look for an oil or concentrate with a more subdued aroma.

Best Pairings: Sour Diesel is the perfect sun-shine strain to enjoy in the open air. Raising the senses to new heights, there's no better companion for days spent on the beach or in the thick of nature.

Recommended Vaping Temperatures:

- 350°F for uplifting mood elevation and creativity
- 390°F for relaxed focus and pronounced euphoria

Indica

Gdp

Grandaddy
Purple

Granddaddy Purple

"Makes me relax hard. I love stretching it out on this strain; I've used this before a massage and before the odd yoga class to great effect. Such a chill euphoria! A great way to wind down in the evening for sure."

King among indicas, this flavorful bud often blooms with beautiful purpled foliage.

Parent Strains: Purple Urkle x Big Bud

Flavors: Sweet red grapes combined with the taste of ripe mixed berries

Description: Introduced in 2003 by Ken Estes, Granddaddy Purple (GDP) is a famous indica born from parent strains Purple Urkle and Big Bud. GDP blooms in shades of deep purple, a contrastive backdrop for its snowlike dusting of white crystal resin. Its potent psychoactive effects are clearly detectable in both mind and body, delivering a fusion of cerebral euphoria and physical relaxation. While your thoughts may float in a dreamy buzz, your body is more likely to find itself fixed in one spot for the duration of GDP's effects.

Consumption Tips: There's no right or wrong way to enjoy Granddaddy Purple, but a vaporizer set to 340°F will best preserve the sweet berry flavor. Find it in oil or edible form to ensure a long, restful night of sleep.

Best Pairings: Few strains pair better with a glass of red wine in the evening. Pull up your comfiest chair to enjoy, or make this indica your bedside nightcap.

Recommended Vaping Temperatures:

- 340°F for relaxing mood elevation
- 395°F for deep sedation

Hybrid

Ww

White Widow

White Widow

"Even after years of daily smoking and vaporizing, this strain's indica side still floors me. [Its] scent and flavor are quite plain and natural, a simple earthen taste with a touch of wood. The first few seconds of a hit will have you calm and relaxed."

The potent and earthy resin-queen hailing from Amsterdam.

Parent Strains: Brazilian sativa x South Indian indica

Flavors: Earthy flavors of sweet wood and hash

Description: Among the most famous strains worldwide is White Widow, a balanced hybrid first bred in the Netherlands by Green House Seeds. A cross between a Brazilian sativa landrace and a resin-heavy South Indian indica, White Widow has blessed nearly every Dutch coffee shop menu since its birth in the 1990s. Its buds are white with crystal resin, warning you of the potent effects to come. A powerful burst of euphoria and energy breaks through immediately, stimulating both conversation and creativity.

Consumption Tips: It's easy to overdo it with White Widow, so dose modestly if you're looking to avoid a premature bedtime. Also, be sure your grinder has a kief catcher, because this one produces a lot of crystal resin.

Best Pairings: A perfect after-work reward, White Widow pairs well with most relaxing activities outdoors or indoors. Fishing trips, campfires, and sunbathing can all be made even more enjoyable with White Widow, or use it after a big dinner to help you relax and digest.

Recommended Vaping Temperatures:

- 330°F for functional relaxation
- 390°F for deep sedation

Bubba Kush

"Effects are classic indica; sleepy, hungry, and happy. A moderate dose results in a feeling just short of couch-lock, allowing you to stay mobile, but at the same time making your chair feel insanely comfortable."

A popular, tranquilizing Kush born and bred in the United States.

Parent Strains: Northern Lights x (OG Kush x unknown indica)

Flavors: A sweet, earthy blend of chocolate and coffee flavors

Description: Bubba Kush is an indica strain that has gained notoriety in the United States and beyond for its heavy tranquilizing effects. Sweet hashish flavors with subtle notes of chocolate and coffee come through on the exhale, delighting the palate as powerful relaxation takes over. From head to toe, muscles ease with heaviness as dreamy euphoria blankets the mind, crushing stress while coercing happy moods. Bubba Kush exhibits a distinctive, bulky bud structure with hues that range from forest green to pale purple.

Consumption Tips: Another THC heavyweight; cannabis novices should ease into this strain slowly. Its chocolate and coffee flavors are best brought out by vaporizers set to about 330°F.

Best Pairings: Arm yourself with Bubba Kush the next time you find yourself battling insomnia, or use it to bring relief to sore, aching muscles. However you choose to kick back with Bubba, just make sure your schedule is clear because you won't be moving much once the effects settle in.

Recommended Vaping Temperatures:

- 330°F for functional relaxation
- 390°F for deep sedation

Pineapple Express

"It helps you forget yourself and unwind. In today's hectic world, it can be your stolen moment to center yourself."

A hybrid strain so good, they made a movie about it.

Parent Strains: Trainwreck x Hawaiian

Flavors: Sweet tropical fruit with a sour pineapple overtone

Description: Pineapple Express combines the potent and flavorful forces of parent strains Trainwreck and Hawaiian. The smell is likened to fresh apple and mango, with a taste of pineapple, pine, and cedar. This hard-hitting sativa provides a long-lasting energetic buzz perfect for productive afternoons and creative escapes.

Consumption Tips: This hybrid's flavor is strong enough to withstand the combustion involved with pipes and bongs, but if you're picky, throw this one in a vaporizer at 350°F to maximize those sweet tropical flavors.

Best Pairings: Pineapple Express's balanced and eclectic nature pairs well with almost every activity imaginable, but nothing is better than sharing this one on a hot summer day. Fresh fruit and citrusy ales are unbeatable companions for this Hawaiian punch of a strain.

Recommended Vaping Temperatures:

- 350°F for uplifting, creative effects
- 390°F for relaxed mind and body

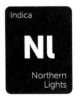

Northern Lights

"Melted into a tub of hot water and listened to music while my thoughts floated away and my body pain dissolved into the bath. The experience developed into a profound sleepiness."

A rumored Pacific Northwest transplant blanketed in starry, crystal-tipped trichomes.

Parent Strains: Afghani x Thai

Flavors: Subtle earthy flavors with an edge of fresh pine

Description: Northern Lights stands among the most famous strains of all time, a powerful indica cherished for its resinous buds, fast flowering, and resilience during growth. Rumor has it that Northern Lights first sprouted near Seattle, Washington, but was propagated out of Holland after 1985 at what is now Sensi Seeds. Northern Lights's psychoactive effects settle in firmly throughout the body, relaxing muscles and pacifying the mind in dreamy euphoria.

Consumption Tips: Powerful euphoria may coerce sleepiness, so however you choose to consume Northern Lights, be sure to do so in the evening or on a lazy day dedicated to doing nothing.

Best Pairings: A jar of Northern Lights may be the only thing standing between you and a good night's sleep. Use this indica as a sleep aid or enjoy it alongside your favorite TV show.

Recommended Vaping Temperatures:

- 340°F for relaxing mood elevation
- 395°F for deep sedation

Sativa
Dp
Durban Poison

Durban Poison

"It wakes you up, cuts through the bleary fog and leaves you clear headed and bright, gives you energy to go and seize the day."

Fuel for focus and creative thought straight from Africa.

Parent Strains: African landrace

Flavors: Earthy spice lifted by the fresh scent of pine

Description: This pure sativa originates from the South African port city of Durban. It has gained notoriety worldwide for its sweet smell and energetic, uplifting effects. Durban Poison is the perfect strain to help you stay productive through a busy day, when exploring the outdoors, or to lend a spark of creativity.

Consumption Tips: Often rich in the rare cannabinoid THCV, vaporize this at 430°F to capture it. THCV is associated with high-energy effects perfect for staying active and focused.

Best Pairings: Durban Poison lights a fire under your creativity, boosting intrigue and engagement in writing, drawing, music, and other creative activities. Grab some coffee and some Durban Poison, and get ready to conquer your to-do list.

Recommended Vaping Temperatures:

- 360°F for uplifting mood elevation
- 430°F for sharp focus and mental stimulation

Strawberry Cough

"I was grinning from ear to ear as I continued to look up at the stars or enjoy the warmth of the fire as this stellar high kicked in . . . keeping me blissfully high for the next two hours."

A sativa that will have you exhaling a lungful of fresh strawberry flavor.

Parent Strains: Unknown

Flavors: Ripe strawberries fresh off the vine

Description: Known for its sweet smell of fresh strawberries and an expanding sensation that can make even the most seasoned consumer cough, Strawberry Cough is a potent sativa blend with mysterious genetic origins. The skunky, berry flavors will capture your senses while the cerebral, uplifting effects provide an aura of euphoria that is sure to leave a smile on your face. Strawberry Cough is a great solution for managing social anxieties and to balance yourself in times of elevated stress.

Consumption Tips: A vaporizer set to about 360°F is the best way to achieve a clean, strawberry flavor, but this strain tastes great in a clean pipe or bong as well.

Best Pairings: Nothing beats a bowl of fresh fruit to quench the dry mouth brought on by this strain from time to time. Social and upbeat, share Strawberry Cough with friends and go on an adventure out in nature.

Recommended Vaping Temperature:

- 360°F for uplifting mood elevation
- 390°F for relaxed focus and pronounced euphoria

Super Silver Haze

"Super Silver just kills depression and evaporates the pressure of stress without turning your mind to mush. It's a very creative, positive high."

A multi-award-winning sativa straight out of Holland.

Parent Strains: Unknown

Flavors: Earthy spice sweetened by orange zest

Description: First bred in Holland and propagated by Green House Seeds out of Amsterdam, Super Silver Haze is a famous sativa known for its energetic, long-lasting high that helps you coast into a positive, relaxed mind-set. A cross between Northern Lights, Skunk, and Haze, Super Silver brings together the best of indica, sativa, and hybrids with an emphasis on the uplifting, weightless sativa effects. It's won numerous Cannabis Cup awards since the late '90s.

Consumption Tips: Super Silver Haze is one of those strains you should have in your back pocket, rolled into a joint or ready to go in your one-hitter. Although it's a great choice for staying productive and uplifted through the day, it tapers into mellow relaxation that can be embraced even late at night.

Best Pairings: Gracefully balancing dreamy introspection with calming physical attributes, Super Silver Haze pairs well with meditation, yoga, and other mindful practices. As it lends a spark to your creativity, you may also try using this strain with your favorite hobby or game.

Recommended Vaping Temperatures:

- 350°F for uplifting mood elevation and creativity
- 390°F for relaxed focus and pronounced euphoria

Indica

Bry

Blueberry

Blueberry

"The only things that top the magnificent blueberry smell are the feelings of relaxation, calm, and focus. It feels like a sativa in many ways except that this can also ease me to sleep if that's what I'm after."

The indica that brought the distinct flavor of blueberry to the cannabis world.

Parent Strains: (Purple Thai x Highland Thai) x Afghani

Flavors: Fresh blueberries bursting from rich soil

Description: The long history of Blueberry is traced back to the late 1970s when legendary American breeder DJ Short was working with a variety of exotic landrace strains. However, throughout the decades of Blueberry's cultivation the genetics have been passed around, due in large part to DJ Short working with multiple seed banks and breeders. The sweet flavors of fresh blueberries combine with relaxing effects to produce a long-lasting sense of euphoria.

Consumption Tips: Blueberry is a great choice for new consumers looking to dip their toe into a gentle indica. Though not totally sedating like many heavy indicas, Blueberry is still preferred for unwinding in the afternoon or evening.

Best Pairings: Use Blueberry as a nightcap before bed, or if you need an afternoon pick-me-up after a long, stressful day. Its flavors pair beautifully with fruity notes of tea and blueberry-based drinks and cocktails.

Recommended Vaping Temperature:

- 340°F for relaxing mood elevation
- 395°F for deep sedation

Hybrid

Che

Cheese

Cheese

"Very strong body high that very much feels as if you're floating in warm water. If you're able to keep completely motionless, you'll feel every muscle in your body slowly [untense] themselves. After a while you won't even want to move, staying in a quiet and still blissful world of your own."

A U.K. strain with unique funky (yep, you guessed it) "cheesy" aroma.

Parent Strains: (Purple Thai x Highland Thai) x Afghani

Flavors: Sharp cheese flavors underlying a pungent earthy coat

Description: Named for its sharply sour aroma, Cheese is an indica-dominant hybrid from the U.K. that has achieved widespread popularity for its unique flavor and consistent potency. With origins that stretch back to the late 1980s, Cheese is said to descend from a Skunk #1 phenotype whose pungent aroma made it stand out. Breeders like Big Buddha Seeds later introduced Afghani indica genetics to increase Cheese's trichome production and yields. The resulting hybrid is now well known for its relaxed, happy effects that gently ease you into a blissful state of mind.

Consumption Tips: Some consumers may be bothered by the unusual aroma of this strain, but if you're embracing the novelty, stick this one in a vaporizer set to 350°F. Using this strain in a bong or pipe will tone down the cheese notes.

Best Pairings: Like the food it takes its name from, Cheese makes a lovely pair with your favorite wine. Combine this relaxing strain with a movie night with friends keeping in mind that conversations shared might not make a whole lot of sense.

Recommended Vaping Temperatures:

- 330°F for functional relaxation
- 390°F for deep relaxation

Hybrid

Ct

Cannatonic

Cannatonic

"I can maintain my energy levels, while grounding myself. Makes me feel more connected to the world, instead of my usual routine of mentally floating around. Best of all, I become more functional and focused."

A CBD-rich variety providing relaxation without the mental fog.

Parent Strains: MK Ultra x G13 Haze

Flavors: Freshly cut wood and earthy soil tinted with sweet citrus

Description: Cannatonic is a unique hybrid strain bred by Spanish seed bank Resin Seeds specifically for its low THC content (rarely above 6 percent) and high CBD content (6 to 17 percent). A cross between a female MK Ultra and a famous G13 Haze male, it produces a relatively short-lived, mellow high that is also uplifting and powerfully relaxing, thanks to the high CBD content. Most phenotypes present with a slight earthy odor and a mild, sweet, vaguely citrusy flavor.

Consumption Tips: Cannatonic is an excellent choice for beginners hoping to ease themselves into cannabis, or for anyone looking for clearheaded relief of stress, anxiety, pain, migraines, and tension. If using a vaporizer, be sure it heats past 356°F to capture Cannatonic's CBD.

Best Pairings: When your to-do list feels too long, look to Cannatonic to help you out. Providing stress relief with only a very mild high, this hybrid motivates productivity without compromising cognition.

Recommended Vaping Temperatures:

- 360°F for clearheaded relaxation and relief
- 390°F for deeper relaxing properties

Hybrid

Acd

ACDC

ACDC

"For someone with crippling anxiety issues that can sometimes drive me to nausea and vomiting, I really can't overstate the amazing feeling of my [symptoms] fading away immediately upon administration of this incredible medicine. For someone like me, CBD has literally given me a new lease on life."

A light footed CBD strain with almost no THC to cloud your mind.

Parent Strains: Cannatonic

Flavors: Fresh forest pine subdued by earthy, woody notes

Description: ACDC is a sativa-dominant phenotype of the high-CBD cannabis strain, Cannatonic. One remarkable characteristic of ACDC is its THC to CBD ratio of 1 to 20, meaning this strain induces no psychoactive effects. Tests have put ACDC's CBD content as high as 19 percent, which helps many patients treat pain, anxiety, epilepsy, multiple sclerosis, and the negative effects of chemotherapy, all without intoxication.

Consumption Tips: A favorite among anxiety sufferers, ACDC is a great strain for anyone sensitive to THC's anxiety-provoking side effects. With vaporizers, note that they should be set to 356°F or higher to ensure CBD is vaporized.

Best Pairings: Social anxiety doesn't stand a chance against the stress-fighting qualities of this head-high-free CBD strain. Use it to keep your cool on hectic days, or as a way to relax muscles while preparing for sleep.

Recommended Vaping Temperatures:

- 360°F for clearheaded relaxation and relief
- 390°F for deeper relaxing properties

Sativa

Tg

Tangie

Tangie

"I get a nice clear uplifted buzz with a blast of mental creativity and charge of philosophic thoughts. Perfect for being outside on a sunny day."

A high-energy sativa strain with unrivaled flavors of sweet citrus.

Parent Strains: California Orange x Skunk hybrid

Flavors: Fresh forest pine subdued by earthy, woody notes

Description: Tangie is another fantastic offering from DNA Genetics in Amsterdam that has quickly gained popularity in its home and is spreading elsewhere. This motivating, cerebrally calming strain is a remake of the popular version of Tangerine Dream that was sought after in the 1990s. The genetics on this strain are a cross of California Orange and a Skunk hybrid, and its citrus heritage is most evident in its refreshing tangerine aroma.

Consumption Tips: Turn that vape up to 360°F and let the sweet citrusy goodness take over. A favorite among flavor fiends and dabbers, Tangie oils and concentrates tend to retain, if not amplify, that pungent orange aroma.

Best Pairings: If you're looking to really spoil your taste buds, pair the sweet clementine flavor of Tangie with citrusy drinks and foods. Uplifting like a warm summer day, take Tangie out for a nature walk and take in the enhanced sights and smells.

Recommended Vaping Temperatures:

- 360°F for uplifting mood elevation
- 390°F for relaxed focus and pronounced euphoria

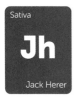

Sativa

Jh

Jack Herer

Jack Herer

"I am unusually vulnerable to feeling anxiety and paranoia when using cannabis, Jack has never even made me tense. A reliable calm and uplifting experience that doesn't cloud my mind."

A Dutch staple delivering mellow euphoria with the uplifting scent of pine.

Parent Strains: Haze hybrid x (Northern Lights #5 x Shiva Skunk)

Flavors: Fresh forest pine subdued by earthy, woody notes

Description: Combining a Haze hybrid with a Northern Lights #5 and Shiva Skunk cross, Sensi Seeds created Jack Herer hoping to capture both the cerebral elevation associated with sativas and the heavy resin production of indicas. Jack Herer was developed in the Netherlands in the mid-1990s, where it was later distributed by Dutch pharmacies as a recognized medical-grade strain. Since then, the spicy, pine-scented sativa has taken home numerous awards for its quality and potency.

Consumption Tips: Jack Herer's gentle euphoria makes this sativa a great choice for new consumers looking for a mellow introduction to cannabis. Vaporizing at lower temperatures will give rise to more clearheaded, alert effects.

Best Pairings: Productive days call for Jack Herer. Whether you're tackling a creative project, cooking, or cleaning, the softly invigorating effects of this sativa should make active mornings and afternoons that much better.

Recommended Vaping Temperatures:

- 330°F for a more clearheaded, focused high
- 360°F for pronounced euphoria and enhanced mood elevation

Lamb's Bread

"This herb really makes me feel energetic but in a good way; no rapid heartbeat, paranoia, or racing thoughts. Just positive energy."

The Jamaican native known to bring thoughtful, peaceful serenity to the mind.

Parent Strains: Unknown Jamaican strains

Flavors: Sharp woody notes mixed with sweet, earthy soil

Description: Lamb's Bread is a bright green and sticky sativa strain. The effects have been known to give mass amounts of energy and positive introspection. Stress subsides quickly with the Lamb's Bread buzz, which can help ease depression. The plant originates from Jamaica, and it's reported that Bob Marley himself encountered this wonderful slice of cannabis genealogy.

Consumption Tips: If you find Lamb's Bread to cause too much activity in the mind, soften the effects by mixing in a high-CBD strain.

Best Pairings: Lamb's Bread has historically been revered for its meditative effects, making it conducive for healing and spiritual practice. It is helpful for getting into a mental flow, and the uplifting tranquility of Lamb's Bread could also assist in exercise and creative escapes.

Recommended Vaping Temperatures:

- 360°F for uplifting mood elevation
- 400°F for sharp focus and pronounced euphoria

Hybrid

Gg4

Gorilla Glue #1

Gorilla Glue #4

"A stress-melting Jacuzzi of bliss to the head and body. This has become my go-to for when I wake on the wrong side of the bed. Almost instant attitude adjustment."

A hybrid with enough stickiness to glue your fingertips together.

Parent Strains: Sour Dubb x Chem's Sister x Chocolate Diesel

Flavors: Pine and fresh garden herbs with a sour, earthy edge

Description: Gorilla Glue #4, developed by GG Strains, is a potent hybrid strain that delivers heavy-handed euphoria and relaxation, leaving you feeling "glued" to the couch. Its chunky, resin-covered buds fill the room with pungent earthy and sour aromas inherited from its parent strains, Chem's Sister (also called Chem Sis), Sour Dubb, and Chocolate Diesel. Taking first place in both the Michigan and Los Angeles 2014 Cannabis Cups as well as the *High Times* Jamaican World Cannabis Cup, this award-winning hybrid's supremacy is no longer a secret, and consumers will search far and wide to get their hands sticky with Gorilla Glue #4.

Consumption Tips: Those new to cannabis should undergo rigorous training before trying Gorilla Glue #4; its THC content regularly passes 20 percent, which may be a bit much for unseasoned consumers. Its stickiness may be useful in joint rolling, but don't take that joint too far away from the couch if you're susceptible to lethargy.

Best Pairings: Gorilla Glue #4 is the perfect strain to stimulate your appetite before a big dinner, or for relaxing with a movie afterward. Potent and long lasting, this hybrid is a best friend to gamers looking to sink a little deeper into their virtual world (and the couch).

Recommended Vaping Temperatures:

- 330°F for uplifting, creative effects
- 395°F for relaxing, sedating effects

Sativa

Mw

Maui Wowie

Maui Wowie

"Smoked a bowl of this and got inspired enough to clean my entire house. I felt incredibly accomplished and rewarded myself by eating a whole chicken. Most active day I've had in a while."

A tropical-tasting sativa straight from the rich soil of Hawaii.

Parent Strains: Unknown Hawaiian strains

Flavors: Sweet tropical fruit with pronounced notes of pineapple, citrus, and papaya

Description: Maui Wowie (not Maui Waui) is a classic sativa whose tropical flavors and stress relieving qualities will float you straight to the shores of Hawaii where this strain was originally born and raised. Since its beginnings in the island's volcanic soil, Maui Wowie has spread across the world to bless us with its sweet pineapple flavors and high-energy euphoria. Lightweight sativa effects allow your mind to drift away to creative escapes, while Maui Wowie's motivating, active effects may be all you need to get outside and enjoy the sun.

Consumption Tips: Consuming this strain is a vacation in itself; enjoy it rolled into a joint or in a readied one-hitter on your next adventure or while relaxing outdoors. Bring your vaporizer to 360°F to harness the full fruity flavors.

Best Pairings: A perfect strain for days spent in the sun, Mowie Wowie's tropical flavors match well with cold fruity drinks and cocktails. The physical energy and motivation brought on by this sativa will encourage you to get outdoors and breathe the fresh air.

Recommended Vaping Temperatures:

- 360°F for uplifting mood elevation and creativity
- 390°F for relaxed focus and pronounced euphoria

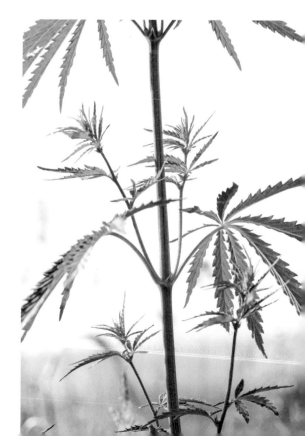

Tips and Strains for Cannabis Beginners

IN MANY INSTANCES, a bad first experience may be enough for someone to banish cannabis from their life forever. More often than not, the reason for doing so has to do with the anxious, paranoid side effects sometimes associated with THC. But what first-timers might not know is that there are a few ways to help minimize and mitigate those unpleasant feelings. For those beginners, lightweights, and low-tolerance consumers, here are three basic tips, tricks, and recommendations for finding that perfect first-time experience.*

* Leafly does not offer legal or medical advice. Any information accessed through the site and services, within any of Leafly's channels, or in this book is for informational and educational purposes only. It is not intended to be a substitute for legal or medical advice, diagnosis, or treatment. Check with your own professionals before using this information.

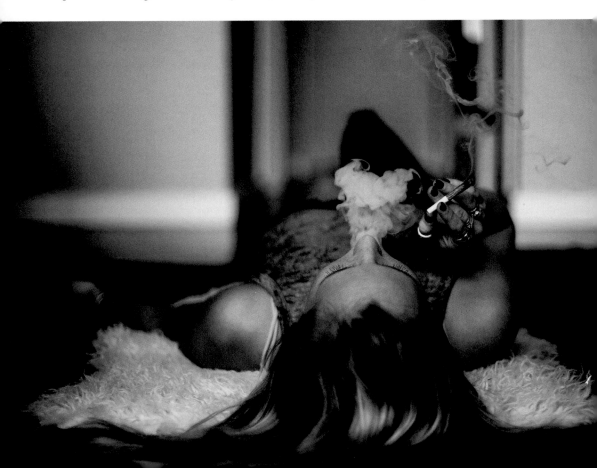

Find a High-CBD Cannabis Strain

Unlike THC, CBD is a nonpsychoactive compound with relaxing and medicinal properties. CBD actually helps counteract the anxiety associated with THC, so it's a perfect starting point for new users. You'll often find strains with equal parts THC and CBD, but some contain almost no THC at all. There are plenty of high-CBD strains around, but here are some of the most commonly found and widely embraced varieties.

COMMON HIGH-CBD STRAINS:

- Harlequin
- Sour Tsunami
- Pennywise
- Harle-Tsu
- ACDC
- Cannatonic
- Canna-Tsu

Start with Low-THC Cannabis Strains

Let's start with the first and most obvious piece of advice: slowly ease into a THC-dominant cannabis strain, as they're more likely to cause anxiety and paranoia. Settle yourself into a comfortable place and start with a low dose, maybe even just a single small hit if it's your first time.

While many strains today tend to stretch toward a THC ceiling of 20 to 25 percent, those with less than 15 percent THC are not as overwhelming. Keep in mind you'll need lab-tested cannabis to know how much THC a flower contains, as amounts can vary between strains and even individual harvests. For example, one batch of Jack Herer may exhibit dramatically lower levels of THC than another, depending on how it was grown and phenotypic variances. Not only that,

there's additional variability that comes with each person's unique brain chemistry and subjective experience.

What works for one beginner may not be the best for the next, but the below recommendations are meant to be starting points for those looking for a more balanced and mellow experience.

HIGH THC STRAINS
WITH A MELLOW HIGH:

- Blue Dream
- Jack Herer
- Chernobyl
- Plushberry
- Maui Wowie
- Permafrost

PRO TIP Have a close friend or partner with plenty of cannabis experience? Ask him or her to help you out if you're nervous— nothing is more comforting than someone you trust close at hand to guide you through the process and allay any apprehension.

Cannabis Delivery Methods Vary in Their Effects

Our advice to you aspiring cannabis champions: Be mindful of the delivery method. The strain is only half of the story; smoking, vaporizing, and ingesting can all affect your overall experience. There's no right or wrong choice here for beginners, but there are nuances between them that should be considered.

Smoking

Most people first try cannabis by smoking it, which has its benefits and drawbacks. One advantage smoking offers is dose control—it's easy to take a small amount and the acute effects usually subside after twenty to thirty minutes. However, the burning sensation in the throat from the first hits may turn some folks off this method entirely.

Vaporizing

Vaporizing may in fact be the most ideal delivery method for newbies. It's gentler on the throat and lungs, dosing is easy, and the flower's flavors are usually better preserved. Portable oil-filled vaporizer pens are a great place to begin since you can take a hit as needed, while tabletop vaporizers give you a larger portion at once, which you'll likely feel obligated to finish (mustn't waste the cannabis!).

PRO TIP For a less intense psychoactive experience, turn your vaporizer to lower temperatures. Try 320°F to 330°F and gradually turn it up if you aren't feeling enough euphoria after a few minutes.

Ingesting

Edibles are a fantastic way to get around smoking cannabis. However, if you're new to the game, start slow and dose low; the effects can take up to an hour or two to kick in, and they tend to be a lot more intense and long-lasting than inhaled cannabis. Cautious consumers may want to start with a tiny dose—maybe just 5 milligrams—and work their way up to the standard 10- to 20-milligram doses.

Topicals

Topicals are cannabis-infused lotions and balms that absorb transdermally for relief of pain, inflammation, and other localized symptoms. Most of them won't get you high at all, so topicals are highly recommended to patients who want medical marijuana without all the cerebral hassle.

What Are the Strongest Cannabis Strains?

WHAT ARE THE strongest cannabis strains? This is a question often asked by consumers with a high tolerance for THC or stubborn medical problems that require a potent product. The answer to this question, however, is a little tricky.

The strongest strains are obviously those with the highest THC content. Generally speaking, anything that surpasses 20 percent could be considered pretty potent. But let's say one grower's harvest of Kosher Kush tested at 22 percent THC. Due to differences in environmental conditions and growing techniques, another grower's Kosher Kush could come out wildly below the mark and test at, let's say, 15 percent.

Even with this variability, there are strains that tend to express higher levels of THC thanks to strong genetics and

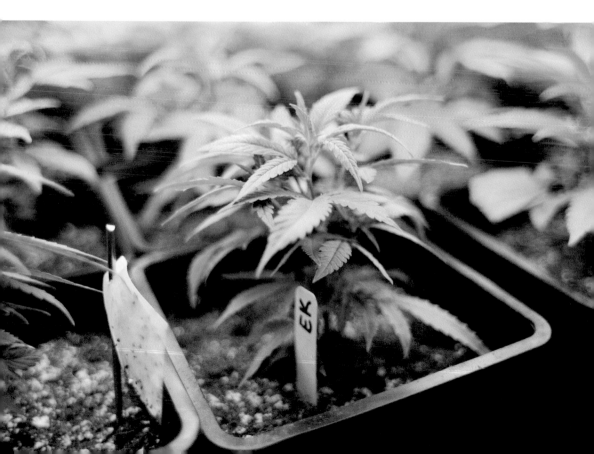

selective breeding. Let's take a look at some of the champion THC heavyweights that have earned awards for their potency as well as some user reviews testifying to their strength.

Girl Scout Cookies

Girl Scout Cookies (no relation to the Girl Scouts, obviously) hauled its way up the ladder of fame in recent years, and it isn't hard to see why. The genetics in this hybrid are strong: according to Steep Hill Labs' data, Girl Scout Cookies typically tests upward to 28 percent THC, and even the low end of its average is a decently impressive 17 percent. The Girl Scout Cookies experience begins with a crushing wave of blissful euphoria, one that enshrouds both mind and body with warm relaxation for hours.

Kosher Kush

Kosher Kush first blessed the world with its presence in 2010 and has been nabbing Cannabis Cup awards ever since. Its genetic background may be a mystery, but this indica's keepers at DNA Genetics have refined a champion strain that consistently breaches 20 percent THC. Wrapped in a thick blanket of crystalline resin, you'll hardly need a closer look to see that this tranquilizing indica is not one for the novices.

PRO TIP Need more potency than flower has to offer? Cannabis concentrates can offer THC heights averaging between 50 and 90 percent, depending on the extraction type and efficiency.

Bruce Banner

Bruce Banner, appropriately named after the Hulk's alter ego—but no relation to the character—is a heavy-duty hybrid with a THC high-water mark of almost 29 percent. Rated the strongest strain in 2014 by *High Times* following its victory in the 2013 Denver Cannabis Cup, Bruce Banner has since carved itself quite the reputation. Powered by OG Kush and Strawberry Diesel genetics, Bruce Banner delivers a dizzying punch of euphoria that anchors your body in deep relaxation.

Ghost Train Haze

In the last few years, the Cannabis Cup leaderboards saw a new rising star: the lively and vigorous sativa known as Ghost Train Haze. Bred by Rare Dankness Seeds, Ghost Train Haze had the highest THC content of any 2011 Cannabis Cup submissions, weighing in at a staggering 25.5 percent THC. Inheriting genetics from Ghost OG and Neville's Wreck, this sativa's potency takes form in a jolt of euphoric energy that goes straight to the head, feeding focus and creativity.

Gorilla Glue #4

Gorilla Glue is named for the stickiness of its resinous buds, and this hybrid certainly lives up to its name. It isn't rare for Gorilla Glue to hit the mid- to upper-twenties in a potency analysis, and it has won multiple Cannabis Cup awards to back that claim up. But we doubt you'll need the proof when this hybrid's got you Gorilla-Glued to the couch in stupefied contentment.

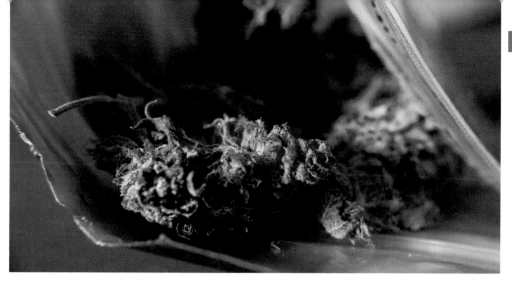

Strawberry Cough

What smells like a bushel of fresh strawberries and has a THC content that'll make even the most seasoned veteran cough? It's Strawberry Cough, winner of numerous Cannabis Cups and the hearts of cannabis enthusiasts around the world. The story goes that Kyle Kushman inherited a really sad-looking mystery clone from a friend's garden and polished it into the sweet-smelling THC engine that now boasts heights of 25 to 26 percent THC content.

The White

Named for the white crystal resin cloaking the buds, the White has become a god-send for breeders looking to improve the potency of their genetics. Routinely testing between 20 and 28 percent THC, the White delivers a disorienting blizzard of euphoric delirium that commands relaxation.

Death Star

With a THC profile that typically dances between 20 and 24 percent, Death Star will surely wreak as much havoc as the Galactic Empire. Using its great psychoactive forces, this Sensi Star and Sour Diesel hybrid commands you to chill out as it imposes powerfully euphoric and sedating effects.

Red Dragon

A Barney's Farm creation, Red Dragon is another familiar name among Cannabis Cup winners. Fiery red hairs shoot out from resin-packed buds, giving this strain a fierce dragonlike appearance. Accurately so, because this strain's path of destruction entails an intoxicating cerebral blast that'll knock bad moods and stress (and possibly common sense) right out.

White Fire OG

Born from the White and Fire OG, White Fire OG (also known as WiFi OG) is a force not to be trifled with. Steep Hill's testing data shows the impressive THC potential of this hybrid, with average levels falling between 22 and 30 percent. Its uplifting effects launch your mood into the clouds, an elevated feeling that will shake your creativity and happiness wide awake.

A Guide to Cannabis Consumption

IN THE MODERN age of cannabis consumption, consumers enjoy a vast array of choices when it comes to partaking. Joints, pipes, bongs, vaporizers, dab rigs, edibles, tinctures, topicals, patches, and many more can all be generalized as means to the same end—and many people lump them together as such. But seasoned consumers know that consumption choice is integral to any cannabis experience.

Preferred consumption methods vary widely, just as reasons for consuming cannabis do. Furthermore, no one method is objectively better than the rest: It all comes down to the goals, preferences, and health concerns of the consumer. An arthritis sufferer uninterested in the psychoactive effects of THC may choose a topical for localized relief, while someone seeking to overcome depression may opt for the euphoria of vaping cannabis flower. Dabbing may send the casual

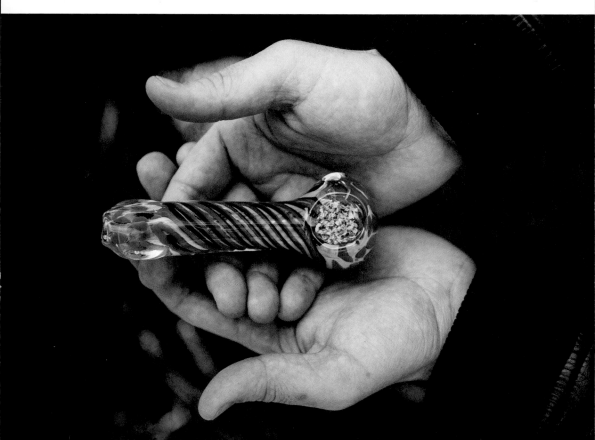

smoker into outer space, but can be a godsend for a cancer patient needing instant relief from chemo-induced nausea. A marathon runner might choose an edible to combat pain and fatigue over long distances. And for friends swapping stories around a campfire, nothing beats the most low-maintenance consumption method of all: the humble joint.

Often, consumers stick to one main method of consumption, but it helps to think of different methods as tools in a toolbox. If you're targeting a single goal day in and day out, you'll likely have a preferred "tool" to get the job done. However, if you use cannabis for multiple reasons, keep your mind open to multiple consumption methods. Need a creativity boost one day? Try vaping a mentally stimulating sativa. The next day, after a trip to the gym, you may prefer a cannabis capsule for muscle soreness.

How to choose the best method for you? Consider your goals, budget, health concerns and personal preferences*. The following overview breaks down the most common basics of each consumption category.

Do one or more of these pique your interest? Read on to dive into the history, nuances, subcategories, and how-tos of each cannabis consumption method in full.

*Consider your comfort in terms of safety. Experiences could vary widely. These methods should only be used in legal states and are done at your own risk.

SMOKING

Benefits: Inexpensive; accessible; classic; social.

Drawbacks: Prohibited in most public places; health concerns; diminished flavor.

VAPING

Benefits: Fast acting; healthy; flavorful; versatile; customizable via temperature control.

Drawbacks: Expensive hardware; not all vapes are portable.

EDIBLES

Benefits: Unique high; body-focused effects; long lasting.

Drawbacks: Slow onset; tricky to dose; doesn't capture strain-specific effects or benefits.

TOPICALS

Benefits: Localized relief; nonpsychoactive; targets CB2 receptors.

Drawbacks: Slow onset; nonpsychoactive.

DABBING

Benefits: Immediate relief; healthier than smoking; works for high-tolerance consumers.

Drawbacks: Difficult to operate; stigmatized; tricky to dose; not for the inexperienced.*

*Hold up: It's time our lawyers step in and tell you a thing or two about dabbing. The amount of heat and fire used in the dabbing process has the potential to be dangerous. Enthusiasts and patients should proceed with caution.

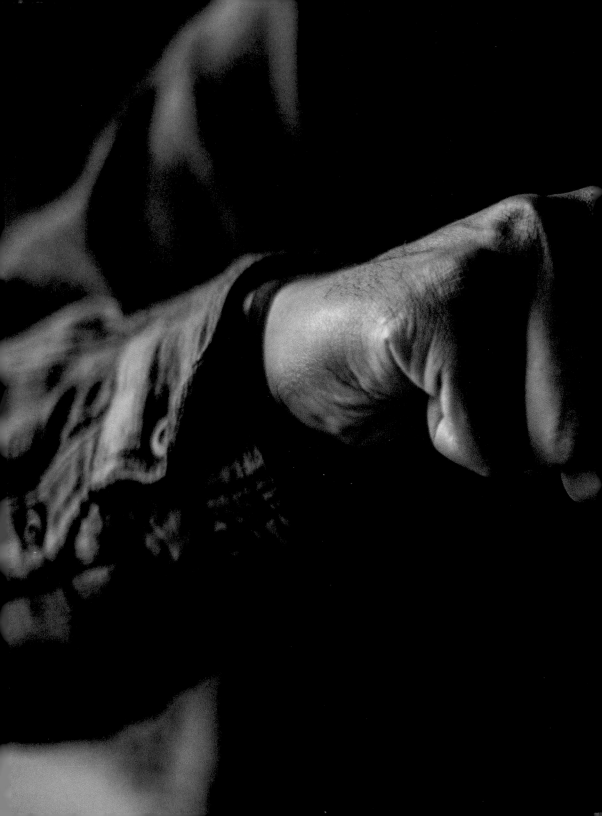

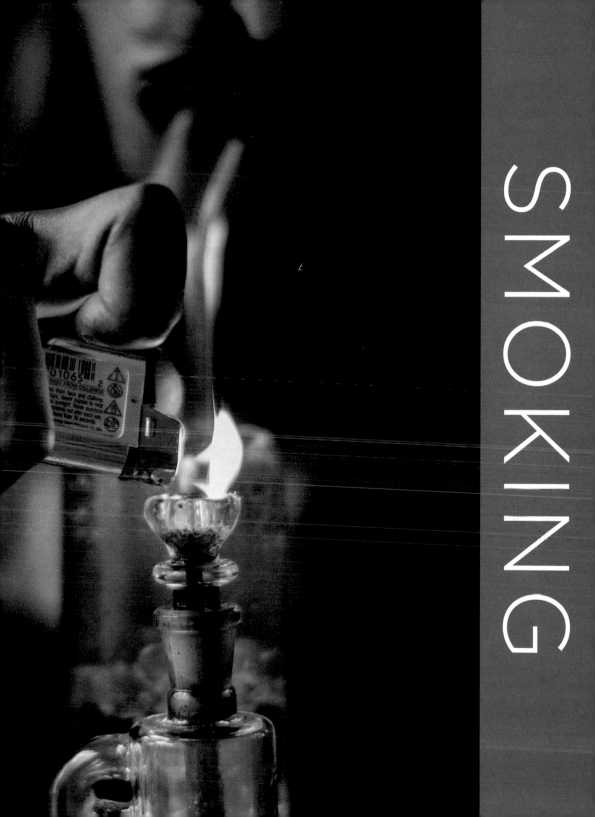

SMOKING

Is Smoking Bad for You?

THE SMOKE ARISING from the combustion of plant material, from any source, contains a lot of toxins and carcinogens. Smoking tobacco cigarettes, smoking cannabis, or sitting near a wood-fueled campfire will all lead to exposure to these substances, resulting in compromised cardiovascular function and other negative health outcomes. Our review of the literature on the health effects of smoking cannabis suggests that cannabis smoke exposure is associated with negative cardiovascular effects and lung function abnormalities, but that the pattern of abnormalities is clearly different from those associated with tobacco smoke exposure.

An area of special concern is whether, like tobacco smoke, cannabis smoke exposure is associated with increased risk of lung cancer (discussed in more detail below). This issue remains controversial, partly due to the inherent difficulty in studying an illegal substance. Because of cannabis's status as a Schedule I controlled substance in the United States, it is much more difficult to conduct the large-scale, high-quality studies needed to fully assess its health impacts. Below is our broad overview of what we know about the effects of cannabis smoke on cardiovascular and lung health.*

*The FDA has not evaluated these effects. Readers should consult their own health professionals and the noted studies themselves.

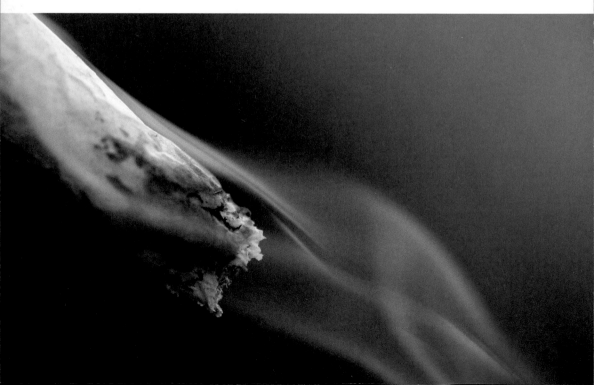

Secondhand Smoke Exposure and Cardiovascular Function

Cardiovascular function is compromised by smoke inhalation of any kind. Recent research has demonstrated that second-hand exposure to cannabis smoke probably impairs cardiovascular function even more than secondhand tobacco smoke. Second-hand smoke exposure impairs blood vessels' ability to dilate. While this has been known for secondhand tobacco smoke exposure for many years, it was only recently demon-strated to be true for secondhand cannabis smoke exposure as well. Moreover, this car-diovascular impairment lasts longer for sec-ondhand cannabis smoke.

It is important to emphasize that the negative effects on cardiovascular function come from the smoke produced by combus-tion of plant biomass and not from inha-lation of plant cannabinoids such as THC or CBD. The cardiovascular impairment described above is observed even when all cannabinoids are removed from the can-nabis used to generate smoke. Because the smoke produced by combustion will always contain toxins and carcinogens, alternative methods of ingestion, such as vaporization, should be considered if one wishes to mini-mize negative health outcomes.

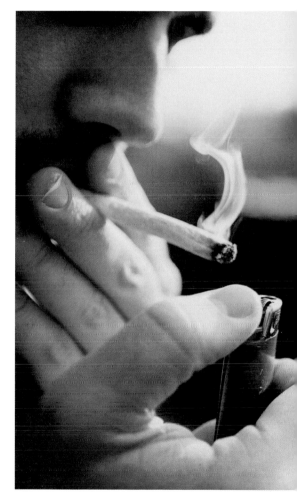

Respiratory Health and Lung Cancer

An extensive literature has documented that tobacco smoke inhalation is strongly linked with increased risk of lung and other cancers. In contrast, there are many fewer studies examining these links with

cannabis smoke, which prevents us from drawing definitive conclusions about can-nabis smoke and cancer risk. Nonetheless, the accumulated evidence so far suggests to us that the risk of lung-related negative health outcomes is far lower for cannabis smoke as compared to tobacco smoke. The reasons for this may have to do with differences between the constituents of tobacco versus cannabis smoke.

Cannabis smoke is like tobacco smoke in that both contain a high number of carcinogens produced by combustion. Certain carcinogens are actually present at higher levels in cannabis smoke compared to tobacco smoke, and cannabis smokers tend to inhale more deeply and hold in smoke for longer durations. Both observations would lead one to expect, if anything, a greater risk of lung cancer for cannabis smoke exposure compared to tobacco smoke. However, this is not the case; a limited number of well-designed epidemiologic studies have failed to find an association between cannabis and increased risk for lung cancer. This apparent paradox may be explained by other differences in the composition of cannabis and tobacco smoke.

Cannabis smoke is different from tobacco smoke in that some of its constituents, such as the plant cannabinoids THC and CBD, are noncarcinogenic and demonstrate anticancer and antioxidant properties. This may explain why several studies have shown no significant link between cannabis smoke and respiratory cancer, at least for light to moderate cannabis smokers. However, there is mixed evidence on cancer risks for heavy, long-term smokers. A few studies have reported an association between cannabis use and upper airway or lung cancers, but these have come from small case-controlled studies that suffered from methodological flaws, such as not accounting for tobacco use. More large-scale studies with rigorous methodologies are needed.

Assessing the effects of smoking cannabis on cancer risk is particularly difficult because cannabis consumption and tobacco use are correlated; the highest-quality studies are those that draw from large samples of individuals and a control for confounding factors such as tobacco use and other variables. While the small number of well-designed population-based studies that have been conducted have generally failed to find an association between cannabis use and lung or upper airway cancer, more high-quality research is sorely needed. Cannabis's status as a federally illegal substance makes this difficult to achieve in a timely fashion.

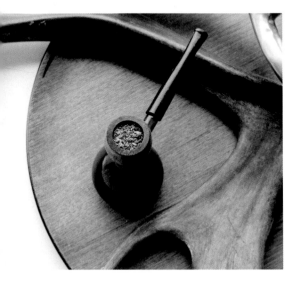

Respiratory Damage and Infection

Another key way that cannabis differs from tobacco is in its effects on the immune system. In general, cannabis has anti-inflammatory and immunosuppressive effects. This may be beneficial for patients suffering from inflammatory diseases such as inflammatory bowel disease or multiple sclerosis. On the other hand, because regular cannabis smoke inhalation causes physical airway damage, the immunosuppressive effects of cannabis may leave regular smokers more susceptible to certain respiratory infections. This is also an area where a greater number of rigorous, large-scale studies would be beneficial.

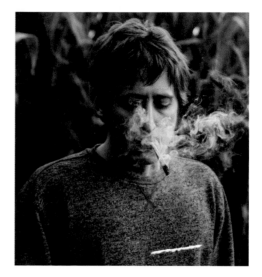

Summary of Potential Cannabis Smoking Risks

Our survey of the scientific literature leads us to conclude the following about the health effects associated with smoking cannabis:

- Overall, the negative effects of smoking cannabis on lung health may be lower than for tobacco smoking.

- Cannabis smoking is associated with lung function abnormalities, but the pattern of these abnormalities is different from those associated with tobacco smoking.

- Regular cannabis smoking can cause physical airway damage, and is associated with the symptoms of bronchitis.

- Secondhand cannabis smoke exposure leads to impairments in cardiovascular function.

- We found no compelling evidence that cannabis smoking leads to obstructive airway disease or emphysema.

- A limited number of high-quality studies have failed to find a link between cannabis smoking and lung or upper airway cancers for occasional or moderate consumers.

- There is mixed evidence for increased cancer risk in heavy, long-term cannabis smokers.

- More research, especially on whether smoking cannabis can lead to lung or other cancers, is desperately needed.

- Alternative methods of cannabis consumption, such as vaporization, do not carry many of the risks associated with smoke inhalation.

How Does a Grinder Work?

GRINDERS CAN BE purchased at almost any smoke store or head shop, or you can order one online from a variety of retail outlets. They can be as simple as a grinding card (like a cheese grater for cannabis) or a more complex multichambered device.* We're going to discuss how to use the most common type of cannabis grinder: a four-piece grinder with a kief catcher. But first, let's go over the basics.

*As cannabis is not legal everywhere, you should check legality before purchasing apparatus.

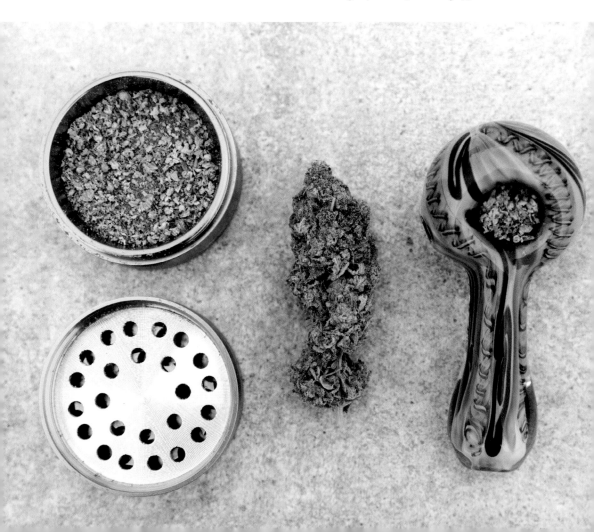

What Is a Grinder and Why Do I Need One for Cannabis?

As you might have guessed, a grinder is the tool you use to break your cannabis up into small bits for smoother-hitting bowls or for wrapping in rolling papers and blunt wraps. There are a number of ways to grind cannabis if you don't have a grinder, but grinders speed up the process and offer perks like kief catchers.

A kief catcher is the bottom chamber below the screen that gathers all the potent crystal kief knocked off the buds in the grinding process. You can scoop the kief out and add it to the top of your bowl, or use it later to press your own hash or cook edibles.

Above the screen, you'll find the grinding chamber with "teeth," or the blades that do all the work. The lid of the grinder attaches to this part, and metal grinders typically have a magnet to help keep things secure as you grind.

How to Use a Grinder

STEP 1:

Take off the top lid. Use your fingers to break up bigger buds and place them in between the grinder's teeth. Don't bother putting any bud in the direct center—this is where the magnet pivots, so nothing in the center will get shredded.

STEP 2:

Replace the top of the grinder and give it about ten rotations, until all the bud has fallen through the holes. You can remove the top and tap it against the grinder's side to help loosen any sticky pieces stuck in the teeth.

STEP 3:

Unscrew the chamber with the teeth to find the basket layer holding all your freshly ground cannabis. Load it into your pipe, joint, or blunt and enjoy!

STEP 4:

Once you've collected kief in the bottom chamber, scrape some out with a piece of paper or the scraping tool provided (not all grinders will include one, but they're definitely handy). Again, you can sprinkle kief onto a bowl to make it more potent, or save it for something else. Be careful with metal scrapers, as they can scrape up aluminum particulates along with your kief.

Some people like to put a weight in the kief chamber to help knock resin from the screen into the bottom dish. A cleaned penny or nickel works perfectly for this.

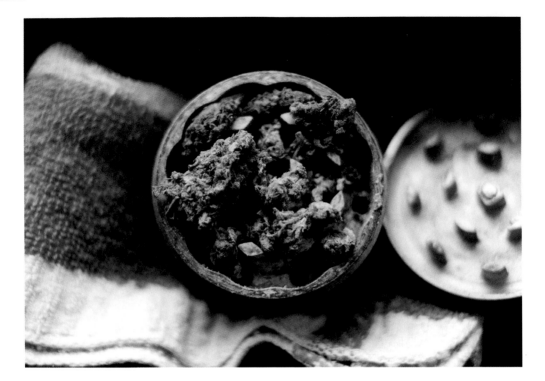

How to Clean a Sticky Grinder

One day, you'll find you have used your grinder so often that it has become sticky with kiefy resin. The threading on the sides where pieces screw together will be gummy, making it difficult (or impossible) to twist open. Avoid having your grinder lock up on you by keeping it clean; here are a few tips for keeping things running smoothly.

- Rub the sticky grinder parts with iso-propyl alcohol and salt. This is a go-to cleaning method for pipes and bongs, but it works just as well for getting rid of the stickiness on grinder pieces.

- Use a small brush (e.g., stiff-bristled paintbrush, clean beard brush, or toothbrush) to knock kief loose from the screen.

- Freezing your grinder makes it harder for kief to stick to surfaces. Consider putting your grinder in the freezer before cleaning up the kiefy mess if it's being particularly stubborn.

- For really irredeemably sticky grinders, sometimes it's best to just replace the thing altogether, especially if it was inexpensive.

10 Ways to Break Up Cannabis If You Don't Have a Grinder

There will come a time when you find yourself without the help of our cylindrical toothed companion, the grinder. Fear not—the ingenuity of a cannabis enthusiast knows no bounds. From simple old school tricks to MacGyver-worthy hacks, here are ten ways to grind cannabis using household items, a bit of creativity, and some care!

1. Your Hands This may seem obvious, but going back to the basics is sometimes the way to go. Plus, this allows you to get up close and personal with your bud.

2. Parchment Pressing To avoid sticky hands, use parchment or wax paper as a barrier between you and your buds.

3. Car Keys Use the serrated edge of a key (after you clean it, of course) to cut away at your buds.

4. Blunt Force When your bud is on the dry side, shake it vigorously in a hard container, or smash a plastic bag against a hard surface.

5. Coin and a Container Drop a clean coin inside of your hard container before giving it a good shake; the coin will thrash around and tear through your buds.

6. Scissors and a Shot Glass Scissors are great for breaking down larger buds, and a shot glass makes a great catching container.

7. Knife and a Cutting Board Pull out a knife and cutting board for a bit of good old-fashioned cannabis carving.

8. Pizza Cutter Like knives, wheeled cutting devices provide a sharp means of slicing.

9. Microplane Microplanes, aka graters, are a perfect alternative to knives, ensuring a fine, even grind.

10. Coffee Grinder A coffee grinder may be the ultimate hack for somebody looking to break down a large amount of cannabis.

How to Pack a Bowl

THERE ARE MANY ways to smoke cannabis, but perhaps none is as well known as smoking a bowl. Learning how to pack and smoke a bowl is a quintessential lesson in cannabis consumption that enthusiasts at every end of the spectrum can benefit from. Whether you're interested in packing a pipe for a personal smoking session or preparing a bowl for a party, understanding these key fundamental principles will help you optimize your experience.

Exploring the Cannabis Pipe

Cannabis smoking contraptions come in all shapes and sizes, but the pipe is arguably the most popular. Adapted from traditional pipes used for tobacco, the cannabis pipe shares all of the same key characteristics. Pipes consist of a "bowl" (thus the popular nickname), which is a round basin deep enough to pack in herbs, and an airtight channel that delivers airflow through a mouthpiece. In many cases, pipes also contain a second air channel known as a carb that is used to ensure the

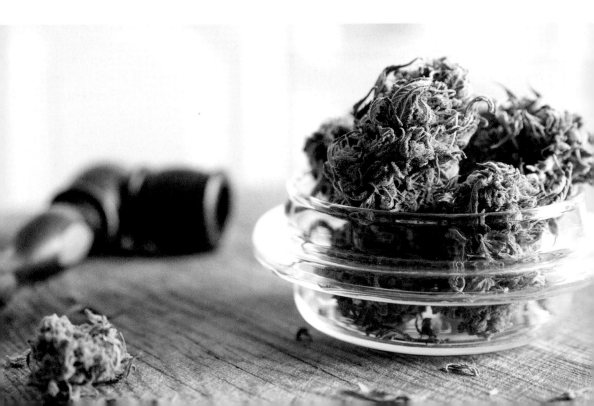

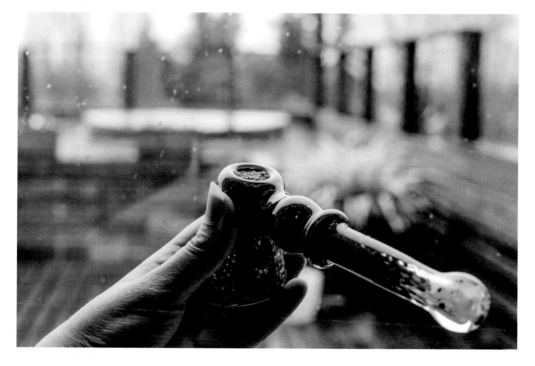

maximum delivery of airflow through the mouthpiece. Some also incorporate water to filter cannabis smoke and cool it prior to inhalation.

Essentially, as long as a pipe includes a bowl and a channel mouthpiece, you can smoke cannabis out of it. The most basic pipes take a physical form many refer to as a spoon. These are the best pipes to begin with if you are new to cannabis, as they are small, easy to use, and are typically inexpensive. However, pipes can vary widely in complexity, functionality, and availability.

Traditionally, pipes used for tobacco-smoking purposes were made out of material such as wood, bamboo, or even ceramics. However, cannabis pipes today are widely made using borosilicate glass, as the medium is incredibly versatile. While glass pipes are still widely marketed as tobacco-smoking devices in most states, they can be found in cannabis and tobacco accessory shops (also referred to as head shops), online, at cannabis events, at medical and adult-use dispensaries, and even in high-end glass art museums.

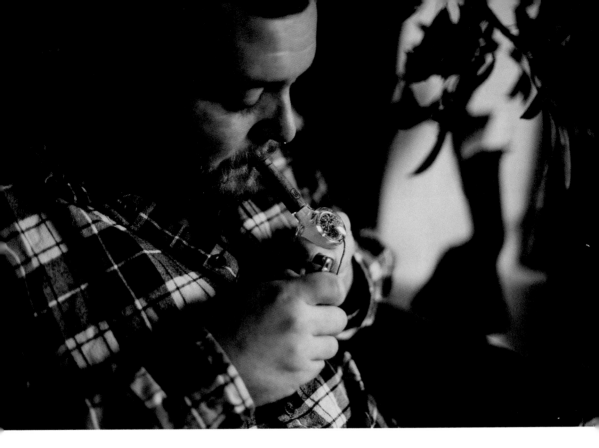

Packing and Smoking Your Bowl

To pack and smoke a bowl, you're going to need a few essential items to get started. In addition to your bowl or pipe, you will need some form of heating element. The most basic heating elements available are matches and lighters. Traditional butane lighters work well, though there is a myriad of non-butane heating elements out there to choose from. The most effective lighters and heaters will allow for optimal heat control when combusting and/or vaporizing a bowl.

Many consumers prefer to light their bowls with hemp wick, a waxy piece of hemp string that ignites easily, maintains an even burn, and doesn't give off an undesirable aftertaste. Another heating element often used is a glass wand that can be heated to a point where it will vaporize your herb on contact, eliminating combustion smoke altogether while still delivering cannabinoids and flavor through a lighter hit.

Preparing cannabis for smoking a bowl is essential in order to maximize airflow through your device and deliver the most even smoke possible. Breaking down your herb is a crucial step: doing so creates a homogenous airflow through the bowl, allowing smoke to pass evenly.

A few tricks that will help to maximize airflow:

1. Ensure that your cannabis is evenly broken down but not too finely ground. Hand pulling your herb is the most basic way to do this, but grinders make the process much easier. There are many ways to break your cannabis down, so don't be afraid to get creative (check out our section on what to do if you don't have a grinder for the details).

2. Use a stem and/or a nice-size intact calyx to stuff at the very bottom of your bowl to prevent particulates from passing though. You can also use a screen if you have one available.

3. Pack your herb very lightly at the bottom and slightly denser at the top for an even smoke. This allows the cannabis toward the top to maintain a burn, or "cherry," while opening airflow for easy inhalation without any clogging.

Follow the Rules of Smoking Cannabis

For everybody first learning how to smoke a pipe, there are a few pieces of etiquette to follow. When smoking with others, make sure to pack a bowl that's proportional to the size of your smoking circle. For an intimate session, packing personal bowls, or "snaps," is great when alone or with another person. This way, you take turns lighting personally packed micro bowls meant to be consumed in one single hit. For larger groups, heavily packed "party bowls" ensure that each smoking buddy gets a fresh hit of green herb.

Traditionally, the provider of the cannabis will decide who is offered the first hit ("greens"). When offered a hit, make sure to only light a fraction of the visible cannabis. This lets everyone get the same great flavor without leaving an ashy hit for somebody. If the bowl is already lit, feel free to pass it, but let your passing buddy know the bowl is "cherried." Lastly, try not to pocket the lighter if it's not yours. Everybody hates a light thief!

Anatomy of a Bong

BONGS ARE ONE of the most common forms of consuming cannabis, especially dried flower. Also known as a water pipe and sometimes referred to by slang terms like "billy," "bing," "binger,"

and more, the bong is so engrained in cannabis culture that many connoisseurs go so far as to name their pieces, turning the otherwise inanimate object into a personality within their smoke circle.

Components of a Bong

The anatomy of a standard bong can be broken down into five basic parts:

Tube

The tube, which ends in the mouthpiece, is the chamber that fills with smoke after it has filtered through the water.

Bowl

The bowl is the bulbous attachment where dried cannabis flower is loaded and combusted. It's often removable, allowing it to function as pull- or slide-carburetor.

Downstem

The downstem is the small tube that allows the smoke to travel from the bowl down to the base, where it percolates through water.

Carb

The carb, short for "carburetor," is a small hole that allows the user to clear smoke from the entire chamber of the bong, completing the bong toke. The most common type of carb found on glass bongs is a pull- or slide-carb, which is exposed when the bowl is removed.

Base

The base is the bottom of a bong and can take many shapes, depending on style. A bubble- or beaker-shaped base is often used to create the water chamber in which the smoke cools as it passes through the water.

TUBE

BOWL

CARB

BASE

DOWNSTEM

All these parts can take various shapes, colors, and designs depending on the bong's intended function. The downstem is often replaced with or attached to a variety of percolator designs that offer more diffusion or separation of the smoke as it passes through the water chamber.

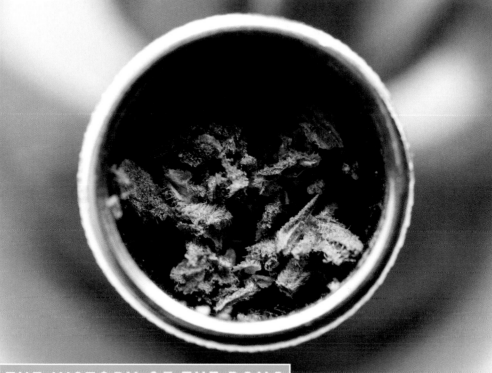

THE HISTORY OF THE BONG

The word "bong" is said to have derived from the Thai word *baung*, which traditionally refers to a round wooden tube of bamboo and in modern Thai is used as the word for a "cylindrical smoking pipe."

Some have traced the use of water in a pipe to filter and cool smoke back to China's Ming dynasty. Other reports show a history of water pipes in Africa, where tribes would build earthen smoking devices into the ground using the same principles behind modern bongs. There are even accounts of bongs made of pure gold used by an ancient nomadic warrior race in what's now modern Russia. Bongs are also closely related to the hookah, a type of water pipe generally used to smoke flavored tobacco. Hookahs use a hose as a mouthpiece and can be designed to allow multiple people to enjoy the smoke from a single bowl.

Today bongs can take on many shapes and sizes, but the most common versions are handblown glass made by artists who blend science and art, creating masterpieces that are both beautiful and functional. This wasn't always the case, though. Throughout its evolution the bong has also been made from a variety of materials, including hand-carved wood, bamboo, ceramic, and even plastic. Many appreciate the MacGyver-like ability to fashion just about anything into a bong, from Coke bottles to watermelons and everything in between.

Cannabis Science 101

The Complex Chemistry of the Bong

WHAT'S GOING ON in that bong? Are those bubbles actually making your toke any healthier? It's complicated. A couple things are happening. Burning cannabis produces a smoke stream that contains all the things you want—activated THC, CBD, other cannabinoids and terpenes—and a lot of things you don't, like hot smoke, tar (a catchall term for the hundreds of nasty compounds produced by cannabis combustion), and fine particulate matter, aka ash.

DID YOU KNOW? Aside from the lack of nicotine, cannabis smoke is qualitatively similar to tobacco smoke, with a lot of polycyclic aromatic hydrocarbons (PAHs) you don't want in your lungs. Too much cannabis smoking can harm the lungs in a number of ways. That said, according to our investigation, despite decades spent looking for one, researchers have not found a link between cannabis smoking and lung cancer.

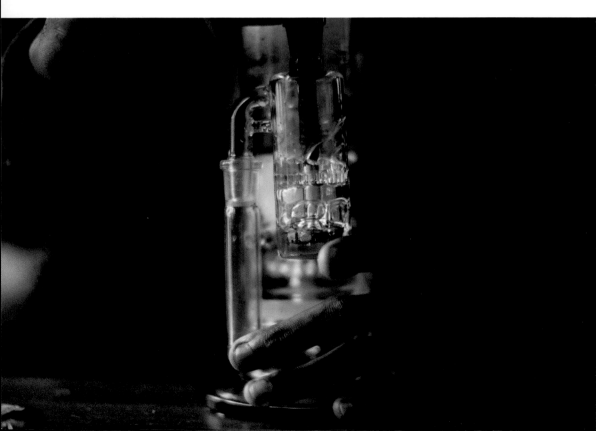

The Filtration Debate

A bong immediately cools each hit by passing it through water, resulting in a smoother toke. The water filters out ash that might otherwise end up in your mouth or airway. There's also a certain amount of tar filtration that goes on. That's why bong water eventually turns sickly brown. There is epidemiologic evidence that tobacco smokers who use a water pipe have a much lower incidence of cancer than those who smoke cigarettes or regular pipes, so clearly this filtration is better than nothing.

That's about the extent of agreement, though. "There's a great debate about whether bongs actually filter effectively," said Kenji Hobbs, manager at Uncle Ike's Pot Shop in Seattle. "Studies in California have shown bongs filter more water-soluble psychoactive cannabinoids than tar and polycarbons, which means the user has to smoke more weed to get an effective high, because the tar-to-cannabinoid ratio is now more skewed towards tar."

Nobody's sure exactly how much cannabinoid filtration might be going on, though. "Those who are familiar with and work in cannabis extractions know that water, as a polar solvent, doesn't do a good job of dissolving cannabinoids, terpenes, or waxes," explained A. J. Fabrizio, director of research for Los Angeles–area medical cannabis company Terra Tech. "Are you losing any cannabinoids or terpenes as the gas passes through water? Yes, but it's negligible. The water will preferentially filter particulate matter and potentially solvate polar molecules, over the cannabinoids and terpenes, which have virtually zero water solubility." This is why cannabis concentrate–makers use nonpolar solvents such as butane, rather than water, to extract cannabinoids from plant matter.

Filtration through a water pipe is not a one-way exchange, though. What's in the water can also change the nature of the smoke. "If you've inhaled through dirty bong water, you know what happens," said Fabrizio. "It tastes like dirty disgusting resin." Further, "if the water has been chlorinated, that chlorine flavor will carry through." That's because the gas is absorbing denatured constituents from the dirty water, such as plant-based molecules that have been fully oxidized during combustion, and that exchange comes through the bubbles. It's a two-way interaction. "This is why people talk about cleaning your bong—and it's also important with dabbing, too. You need to make sure that chamber and that water is pretty clean if you want to ensure an unadulterated flavor."

Optimizing the Water Pipe

A gas-liquid exchange occurs only between the surface area of each bubble and the surrounding liquid in a bong. "Really big bubbles offer relatively low surface-area-to-volume ratios," Fabrizio explained. "A diffuser that produces a lot of smaller bubbles offers a relatively high surface-area-to-volume ratio, allowing for greater exchange between the gas and liquid," and presumably a greater degree of filtration.

Does it make sense to use alcohol—vodka or similar—in the chamber? "Not advised, or safe," cautioned Fabrizio. "Huffing alcohol fumes is toxic." In addition, cannabinoids and terpenes are more likely to dissolve in alcohol than water, so you're essentially stripping the smoke of its more desirable compounds. It's also a nasty inhalation experience.

Very few studies have been done on cannabis and water pipes, and those studies have turned up curious data. That "California study" Hobbs of Uncle Ike's referred to was carried out in the mid-1990s by Dale Gieringer, NORML's California state coordinator, in association with MAPS, the Multidisciplinary Association for Psychedelic Studies. They wanted to test the effectiveness of bongs, joints, and vaporizers. They found that unfiltered joints actually outperformed the bong—by quite a lot. The bong, they reported, "produced 30 percent more tar per cannabinoids than the unfiltered joint." The vaporizer—at the time, one of the earliest on the market—vastly outperformed them all, delivering far more cannabinoids per unit of tar.

One of the problems, Gieringer wrote

back then, was that the researchers were forced to use poor-quality marijuana supplied by the National Institute on Drug Abuse, with THC levels of 2.3 percent. (Today's legal cannabis typically ranges between 15 to 25 percent THC.) That little detail matters, because it requires consumers to burn more leaf—and inhale more unwanted by-products—to obtain the desired level of cannabinoid intake. "We were surprised and a little disappointed at the time," Gieringer recalled. "But we learned that vaporization looked good, even with what was at the time a really crude device."

Also in the mid-1990s, University of Wisconsin pharmacologist Nicholas V. Cozzi penned a literature review of past water pipe studies, mostly from the 1960s and 1970s. He found that the devices "can be effective in removing components from marijuana smoke that are known toxicants, while allowing the THC to pass through relatively intact."

The conflicting results were puzzling, to say the least, and pointed out the need for further study. Unfortunately, further water pipe studies were not forthcoming. Researchers instead focused their attention on studies of vaporizers as a healthier vehicle for cannabis dosing. In the meantime, Gieringer had a tip for those looking for a healthier form of intake: Consider more cannabinoids per unit of vegetable matter.

"The easiest way for most smokers to avoid harmful smoke toxins," he wrote, "may be simply to smoke stronger marijuana."

Advantages of Smoking from a Bong

The main advantage that draws people to using a bong is its ability to cool and filter the smoke through water, offering a smooth draw even when a large amount of smoke is inhaled. When compared to alternative consumption methods, the other advantages can vary.

For those who typically roll their cannabis into joints, bongs offer cooling percolation while maintaining the pungent spectrum of aroma and flavor that cannabis produces. Compared to a standard dry pipe, the bong usually results in a much smoother toke that is less harsh and easier on the throat and lungs than the pipe's hot, dry heat. Bubblers, on the other hand, offer the portability of a hand pipe with the added functionality of water percolation. However, a bong tends to be a more fluid experience than a bubbler, offering less trouble than a bubbler's smaller components, which can often get clogged or dirty.

What Happens When You Replace Bong Water with Something Else?

It's one of those "high-deas" many cannabis consumers have had: How does switching in a different liquid for the water in your bong change the flavor and effects of the resulting hit? Does it make it better? Does it even make a difference? Answer: It depends what you substitute.

We asked the Leafly community to share the strangest things they'd tried subbing in for bong water. Answers included (and were certainly not limited to):

- Soda
- Fruit juice
- Tea (hot or iced)
- Frozen strawberries
- Gatorade (partly for festive color)
- Water with eucalyptus oil
- Snow
- Chicken broth
- Milkshakes
- Mouthwash
- Skim milk with rosewater
- Chocolate pudding
- Alcohol (*strongly discouraged*)

The Leafly team's personal favorite? Soda water with lime.

Joints, Blunts, and Spliffs

What's the Difference?

THERE ARE THREE broad categories by which to delineate rolls: joints (marijuana cigarettes), blunts, and spliffs. Each type of roll can be defined by the content of the roll as well as by the wrapping material used to craft them. While edibles, vaporizers, and dab rigs have all gained popularity as alternative means of cannabis consumption in recent years, the minimalist, easily accessible, tried-and-true art of rolling still reigns supreme globally, and the creative potential and skill required to craft a functional roll is celebrated among many cannabis enthusiasts.

What's Inside Them?

Joints and blunts contain only cannabis. That said, blunts are rolled with tobacco paper (distinguishable by thickness, weight, and dark brown color), whereas joints are rolled with lighter, partially translucent papers. Joints often include a paper filter known as a crutch, which adds stability to the roll and allows you to enjoy your joint all the way to the end, without burning your fingertips. Spliffs

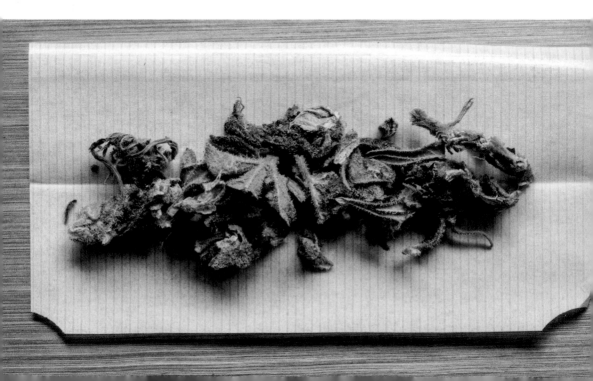

contain a mix of cannabis and tobacco. They're rolled in the same types of papers as joints and also often include a crutch.

The three rolls most notably differ by experience. Tobacco provides an initial head rush and energetic physical buzz (similar to caffeine), which precede the effects of cannabis. This sensation is most notable in spliffs thanks to the presence of loose tobacco. Blunts are generally considered to be the heaviest hitters due to the interaction between the tobacco paper and the cannabis; the added buzz from the paper will either balance the relaxing effects of indica strains or augment the uplifting effects of sativa strains.

The Paper Difference

Paper choice is paramount to your smoking experience, impacting the amount of cannabis used (contingent on paper size), flavor (tobacco papers are notably sweeter than other types, such as hemp paper), and burn (thicker papers tend to burn more slowly than thinner papers). Consumers utilize loose papers to roll joints and can use either loose papers or pre-rolled cigarettes to make spliffs (with the latter requiring careful deconstruction to keep the paper intact).

The aromatic potency of the paper is pertinent for all rolls. Some consumers believe that flavorful papers meddle with the complex aromas of cannabis, while others grow loyal to specific brands thanks to their distinct flavors (this is common among blunt aficionados, who tend to cherish the sweetness of certain tobacco papers over others).

Consumers also choose papers based on rolling ease and functionality. The best papers don't tear, seal seamlessly, handle well between your fingers, and burn uniformly. Nothing is a surer sign of a failed roll than a joint that "runs" (i.e., burns lengthwise along one side).

Regional Preferences of Joints, Blunts, and Spliffs

The popularity of joints, blunts, and spliffs varies regionally, reflective of cannabis culture across the globe. Spliffs are predominant in Europe, where joints are commonly seen as "wasteful"—however, this may change as cannabis prevalence and accessibility rises. Consumers in the United States are more inclined to roll joints than spliffs, possibly due in part to widespread awareness of the adverse health effects of tobacco.

Global differences in terminology are also interesting to note. In Europe, for example, the names are reversed: A joint refers to a roll with cannabis and tobacco (because a "joint" is a combination of two items), whereas a spliff refers exclusively to rolled cannabis.

Finally, it's important to note that joints, spliffs, and blunts are only the beginning. The landscape is expansive, and even within these three delineations, the room for artistic creation is vast.

A Brief History of the Joint

WHILE HUMANS HAVE been consuming cannabis for thousands of years, it has historically been smoked through a pipe, hookah, or chillum. A relatively new innovation, the humble marijuana cigarette has managed to find its way into the heart of countless cultures around the world. Here's a brief overview of its rise to fame.

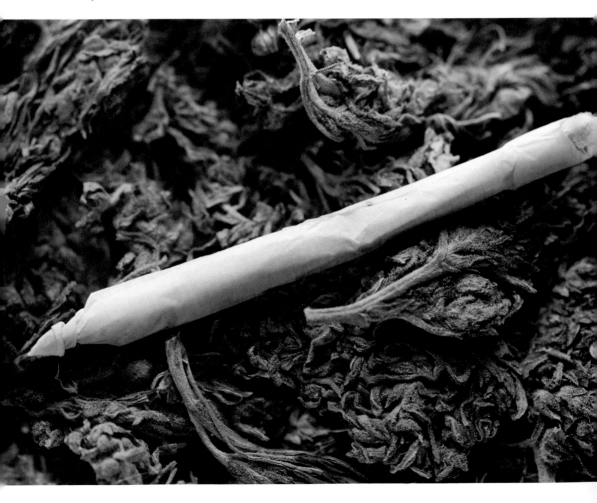

Joints in the Early Twentieth Century

Spurred on by the precursor of Marcus Garvey's Rastafarian movement, cannabis gained a more widespread popularity throughout black communities. Jazz musicians especially preferred cannabis to alcohol, as it enhanced creativity without affecting their motor control.

Many nicknames for cannabis cigarettes were birthed in the '20s and '30s, some of which are still used to this day. The words "reefer" and "joint" originated in this era, as did the term "muggle," since popularized by the Harry Potter franchise (with a completely different meaning). Some words haven't stood the test of time so well. Ever heard of a killer, goof butt, or joy smoke?

The U.S. prohibition of alcohol in 1920 had a big hand in cannabis's widespread usage. Speakeasies were springing up around the country, providing an illegal underground hub where patrons could sip on the finest bathtub whiskey and listen to jazz. New Orleans musicians began touring the country, bringing with them their iconic "jazz cigarettes." Popularity of the drug boomed--its legal status in most states meant that a viper (the term for a cannabis smoker) could roll a reefer in public and face no repercussions.

After a series of increased restrictions and *Reefer Madness*–style propaganda, the Marihuana Tax Act of 1937 was passed federally, essentially outlawing the possession and sale of the plant. Joints were especially targeted in the media, with newspapers and even school textbooks from this era claiming that harmless cigarettes were being spiked with cannabis in order to drug children and drive them insane.

When Was the First Joint Consumed Recreationally?

The first recorded use of a joint was in Mexico in 1856 (although, of course, it probably started much earlier than this). Though cannabis had been used as a medicine for a long time, it seems that the joint was first used for recreational purposes. It was a pharmacist at the University of Guadalajara who first mentioned that laborers were mixing cannabis with tobacco in their cigarettes.

You don't have to look far to spot the cultural ties that still linger from cannabis's Mexican roots. In fact, the word "roach" got its name from the Mexican song "La Cucaracha," which tells the story of a cockroach who can't get up because he has no marijuana to smoke.

The earliest record of a commercial cannabis cigarette can be found in an 1870 publication of *The Boston Medical and Surgical Journal*. Grimault's Indian Cigarettes—marketed as a treatment for respiratory ailments—were a powerful mixture of cannabis resin, belladonna leaves (also known as deadly nightshade, a powerful and sometimes lethal muscle relaxant), and a small amount of potassium nitrate. This combination would have acted to expand the bronchial tubes in the event of an asthma attack, allowing the patient to increase oxygen flow to the lungs.

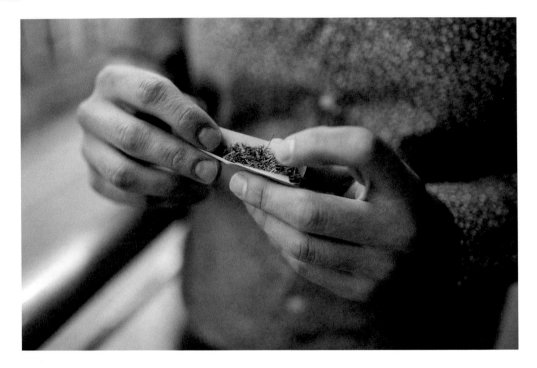

Popularity of "Marijuana Cigarettes" Skyrockets

The 1960s marked a major shift in people's attitudes toward authority. The conflict in Vietnam was gaining a reputation as an unjust war, and adults who had been raised to believe *Reefer Madness* propaganda realized they had been deceived. Cannabis was not a plant that drove people to homicidal madness, nor would it make a person see demons or become a sex-crazed maniac. Smoking a joint came to represent an act of nonviolent protest against a broken system, and brought people together under the banner of peace, love, and a countercultural revolution.

Hippies were quick to develop their own fashion trends, with many accessories being targeted to stoners. Jewelry and belt buckles were manufactured to include disguised roach clips, allowing the average toker to always be prepared for a surprise spliff, and giving a nod to those in the know.

Rolling paper manufacturers were quick to cash in on this new market, too. Companies created wider styles of papers to accommodate stoners, who traditionally rolled much thicker cigarettes than tobacco users. Packets of rolling paper were decorated with psychedelic patterns and pro-marijuana quotes. A company called Randy's even invented the Insta-Roach wired rolling papers, which gave users a stainless steel wire to hold on to as they finished off the last of their joint.

Cannabis became popular in some pretty unlikely places. Soldiers in Vietnam smoked pot in previously unheard of quantities, with some commanders asserting that 70 to 80 percent of their troops had tried it. Cannabis usage was an open secret on many bases, with some officers even allowing under-the-counter sales of joints at PX facilities. For just two dollars, a soldier could buy a packet of real cigarettes that had been emptied out and filled with cannabis. Many even had the original cellophane seal reapplied. Discreet and unassuming, these disguised doobies became especially useful when the military decided to search your quarters.

Modern-Day Joints

Today, although cannabis remains illegal federally and in many states, its use and distribution is legal in an increasing number of states for medical purposes, and, in some states, for adult recreational use. These discerning cannabis connoisseurs in legal states can customize their rolling experience to a degree that has never been seen before. Legal consumers can choose from a huge selection of strains, treat themselves to special papers, and even purchase power packed pre-rolls. Thanks to the Internet, we're also starting to see some incredible art emerge from professional joint rollers, such as Tony Greenhand, one of the biggest pro rollers on the scene.

Simple, convenient, and time honored, it's easy to appreciate a joint.

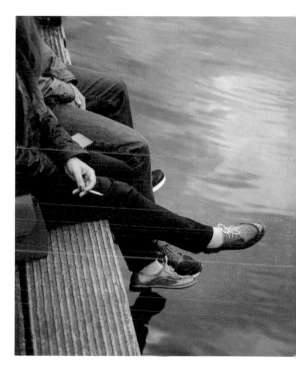

The Science of Joints

WHEN A JOINT gets passed around, it tends to bring out the armchair scientists. Everyone has a theory. And most theories sound like they come straight from the mind of Ron Slater, the stoner historian in *Dazed and Confused.* There's the temperature theorist, who's convinced you've got to keep the joint hot. And the long-toke artist. And the many-short-hits believer. But who's right?

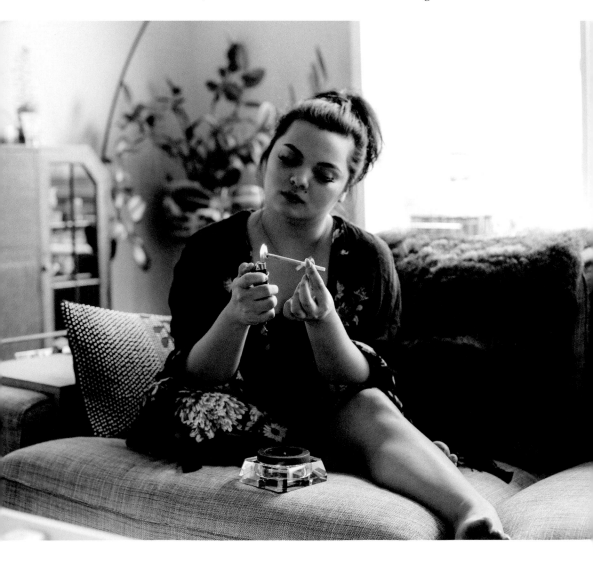

Why We Smoke It

First, some information about why cannabis is burned and smoked in the first place. Eating a gram of cured flower straight out of the bag is a bad idea. It'll taste like eating Kentucky bluegrass, and you won't get the desired effect. The THC in the plant needs to undergo a process known as decarboxylation to become psychoactively available. Ed Rosenthal, one of the world's leading experts on cannabis biology, explains the rest in this excerpt from one of his columns:

Marijuana produces THCA, an acid with the carboxylic group (COOH) attached. In its acid form, THC is not very active. It is only when the carboxyl group is removed that THC becomes psychoactive. When marijuana is smoked, the THC behind the hot spot is vaporized as the hot air from the burn is drawn through the joint or pipe bowl to the unburned material.

How Much THC Moves from Leaf to Bloodstream?

One of the earliest NIDA (National Institute on Drug Abuse) studies on cannabis cigarettes, conducted in 1982 by NIDA researcher Richard L. Hawks, estimated that 20 percent of the THC in a cannabis cigarette was delivered to the body when the smoker took a five-second puff each minute. All the rest was lost to pyrolysis (burning) and sidestream smoke (the stuff rising from the smoldering end).

A later study in 1990 by Mario Perez-Reyes, a psychiatric researcher at the University of North Carolina, put more specific figures to the path taken by THC. He estimated that 20 to 37 percent of the THC in a joint hits the consumer in mainstream smoke. Twenty-three to 30 percent is lost to pyrolytic destruction, and 40 to 50 percent goes up in sidestream smoke.

In these early studies, the scientific concern was all about THC. Other cannabinoids, like cannabidiol (CBD), and terpenes weren't yet widely known. Also worth noting. All of these American studies were conducted using low-quality, low-potency (1.5 to 3 percent THC) cannabis supplied by NIDA.

Those estimates allow us to run some interesting numbers. If the average joint contains about 700 milligrams of cannabis flower—that's the "scientific test joint" configuration—and today's average THC level runs around 20 percent, that means 140 milligrams of THC are available in each joint. If 20 to 37 percent of that carries to the lungs, that's a THC dose of 28 to 52 milligrams. Before you start comparing that to THC milligrams in edibles, though, consider that the body metabolizes and reacts to edibles differently than it does to inhaled smoke.

More Short Puffs, or Fewer Long Draws?

A 2008 study conducted by researchers at Leiden University in the Netherlands, using much better cannabis (17.4 percent THC) supplied by Bedrocan, the company that grows pharmacy-grade cannabis for the Dutch Ministry of Health, specifically tested the toke question. Using joints with 700 milligrams of flower, volunteers tried a puff every which way. They took a two-second pull every fifteen seconds, then every thirty seconds, then every sixty. They tried a two-second pull, a three-second pull, and a four. Then the researchers drew blood from the subjects and measured their plasma THC levels. THC levels in the blood stair-stepped, as expected, in nearly every case. In other words, a longer toke drew more THC into the blood. A greater volume of inhaled smoke did the same.

But here's the interesting thing: The short, two-second puff every thirty seconds and every sixty seconds yielded about the same amount of THC, around 22 nanograms per milliliter (ng/ml). But the same puff every fifteen seconds doubled the THC intake, to 44 ng/ml.

The conclusion: The average overall temperature of the joint remained higher when a toke was taken every fifteen seconds. That kept the whole THC decarboxylation and delivery system up and running. When the joint was allowed to rest for thirty or sixty seconds, it cooled. It's the difference between keeping a machine running and or shutting it down and starting it back up again. Plus, as a number of these study authors noted, cannabis cigarettes don't burn nearly as evenly or well as tobacco cigarettes. If you leave them untended for too long, they have a tendency to extinguish themselves.

Perez-Reyes observed a similar dynamic during his 1990 study. He asked study subjects to smoke joints extremely fast—a hit every six seconds—and then more slowly, taking a drag every seventeen seconds, which is still pretty fast. And his subjects got really high. The six-second-interval smokers registered peak THC blood plasma levels of 210 to 230 ng/ml. The seventeen-second-interval smokers hit 100 to 160 ng/ml. The legal limit for impaired driving in both Washington and Colorado is 5 ng/ml.

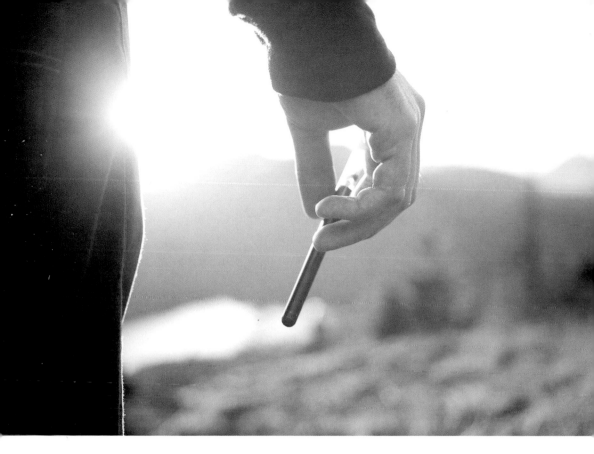

Delivery Efficiency: Joint vs. Vape vs. Bong

In 2007, Donald Abrams, a pioneering medical cannabis researcher at the University of California, San Francisco, published a study of THC intake via the Volcano-brand vaporizer. Abrams tested the vaporizer as a safer alternative to cannabis cigarettes. He was responding to a 1999 Institute of Medicine report that found medical value in cannabis but hedged against recommending medical marijuana "because of the health risks associated with smoking."

Abrams did find vaporization to be healthier. Compared to a smoked joint, the Volcano produced far less tar, carbon monoxide, and other combustion by-products while delivering almost identical blood THC levels. The vaporizer captured 54 percent of the THC in the leaf, as compared to the 20 to 37 percent available from a joint.

Bongs, by comparison, may deliver less THC per gram of flower. Perez-Reyes found that peak blood THC levels among his subjects using a water pipe were about 50 percent lower than the blood THC levels among the same subjects smoking the same amount of cannabis in a joint. That finding may lend credence to those who wonder if bong water is filtering out some of the cannabinoids that consumers desire.

Self-Titration Is a Real Thing

For UCSF's Donald Abrams, the most surprising data from his 2007 study may have come in the area of titration—a factor involving concentrations of THC in the blood (more later). He asked his subjects to consume three different potencies: 1.7 percent THC, 3.4 percent, and 6.8 percent. Under perfect conditions, the blood THC levels of the subjects should have stair-stepped along with the increased potencies. But they didn't.

Smoking the 1.7 percent THC cannabis, his volunteers peaked at blood THC levels of 80 ng/ml. At double the leaf potency (3.4 percent THC), they peaked at 110 ng/ml. And at four times the potency (6.8 percent), they peaked at 120 ng/ml.

Even though the Volcano captured a higher percentage of THC compared to a joint, blood plasma THC levels in the subjects using those devices were comparable.

Here's the really interesting part: Subjects in Abrams's study didn't know the THC content when they were consuming.

That suggests that the study subjects carried out some sort of self-titration, whether they were aware of it or not. "Titration" is a fancy word for dosing. Self-titration means smokers adapt their smoking behavior to obtain desired levels of THC from the particular delivery system, taking more puffs and/or inhaling more efficiently at lower, compared to higher, THC strengths. "The phenomenon of self-titration of psychoactive drug intake from an inhaled delivery system is well documented for nicotine from cigarette smoking," Abrams wrote, "but to our knowledge has not been previously reported for marijuana."

Abrams's study has interesting policy implications as well. One of the arguments used against recreational legalization is the fear that today's higher-THC cannabis is not the pot you knew in the 1970s. That's true. But it may also be true that consumers are simply inhaling less smoke or vapor than they did in the '70s to achieve similar results.

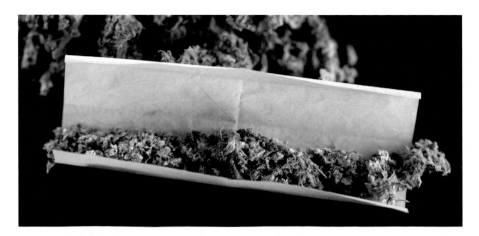

Step by Step

How to Roll a Perfect Joint

THE JOINT IS one of the more iconic ways to consume cannabis, and every cannabis smoker should learn how to roll a joint that burns smoothly and evenly. Begin by gathering your rolling supplies:

- Cannabis strain of your choice (the average joint contains about half a gram of flower)
- Rolling papers
- Crutch (filter) material such as an index card (optional)
- Cannabis grinder

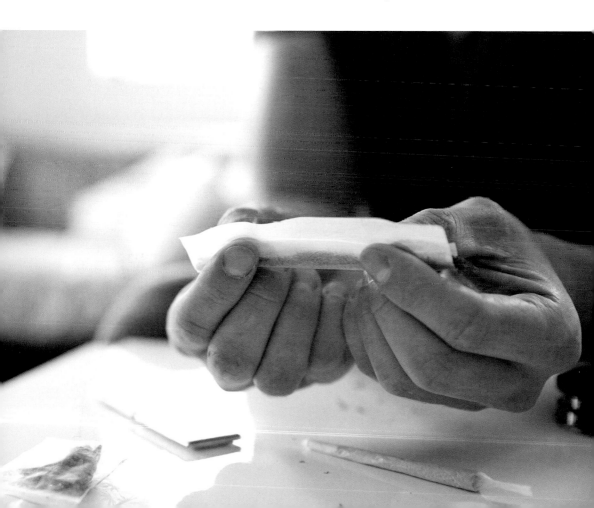

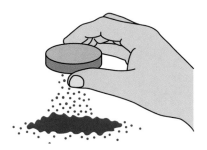

Step 1: Grind the Cannabis

Break down your cannabis into shake. If your cannabis was dried well, it should break down easily. A grinder keeps your hand from getting sticky and thus sticking to the joint paper, but if you don't have a grinder, you can break the herb down by hand, using scissors, or in any other way (refer to our chapter on grinder substitutes for details).

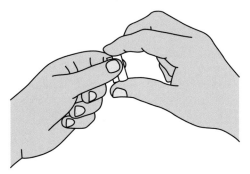

Step 2: Create the Crutch

Make a crutch, also called a tip or filter. You can make a crutch out of just about anything, but cardstock products, such as index cards or business cards, are solid go-tos (though try to avoid any with shiny printing or plastic coating). A lot of joint papers also include crutch material with their packaging.

Cut a thin strip (half inch to one inch wide and at least a couple inches long) of the cardstock material. Start with a few "accordion" folds at one end of the cardboard, then roll the remaining material around the folds to reach the desired thickness of your joint. The crutch isn't absolutely necessary, but it does help keep the shake from falling out of the end or into your mouth as you smoke. It also adds some stability to the joint and allows you to enjoy every bit of cannabis without burning your fingertips.

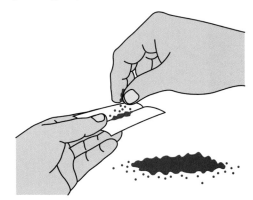

Step 3: Fill the Joint Paper

Set the joint paper, which comes folded lengthwise, in front of you. You'll notice that one edge of the paper has been preglued—make sure this shiny edge is on the far side of the paper, facing toward you. Place the crutch (if you've made one) at one edge of the folded paper, then fill the remaining paper with your ground cannabis.

A quick note on papers: There are a lot of different types and flavors of joint papers available. Many people prefer hemp papers because they tend to be thin but strong, and burn evenly without affecting the flavor of the cannabis.

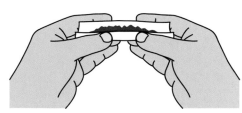

Step 4: Shape the Joint

Once you've loaded your joint, you can begin to form and shape the joint with your fingers. Pinch the paper between your fingertips and roll it back and forth to pack the cannabis down into its final shape.

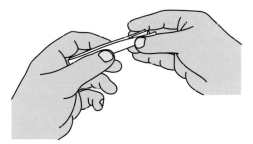

Step 5: Roll the Joint

This step can make or break the quality of your joint. As you pinch the paper between your fingertips, tuck the unglued side of the paper (the side closest to you) over the packed cannabis and into the roll. Roll the glued edge over the unglued edge to tack down one end of the joint, using just a bit of moisture (e.g., lightly licking the paper) to seal it.

Once the paper is tacked on one end, you can work your way down the rest of the seam by tucking and sealing the joint from end to end.

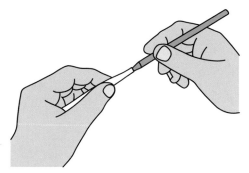

Step 6: Finish Your Joint

Finally, pack the cannabis down from the end of the joint to help ensure an even burn. A pen or pencil works great, but you can use just about anything. Some good options if you're on the go: the tip of your shoelace or drawstring on your hoodie, or a small stick.

If you're not planning on sparking your joint right away, close the tip with a twist to keep the cannabis from spilling out.

Step 7: Enjoy (and Innovate!)

There are Innumerable ways to roll a joint. Joints can be big or small, straight or tapered, featuring multiple connected rolls (like a cross joint) or a single, pristine cone that showcases your dexterity and precision. Get creative! Over the years, masterful rollers have transformed joint rolling into an art form all its own.

Step by Step

How to Roll a Perfect Blunt

A BLUNT IS to a joint what the cigar is to a cigarette; or more simply, it is a cigar that has been emptied of its loose-leaf tobacco and filled with cannabis.

While not quite as iconic as the standard joint, the cultural significance of the blunt cannot be ignored. Many enjoy the buzz imparted by the mix of cannabis and its tobacco wrap, while others appreciate the variety of flavors available in most cigarillos and blunt wraps.

Rolling a blunt comes with its own set of norms that are in place to maintain function and tradition. To roll up your own, start by gathering the necessary supplies:

- Cannabis strain of choice (average blunts contain two to three grams of flower)
- Cigar, cigarillo, or blunt wrap
- Grinder and blade (optional, but may be helpful for those new to rolling)

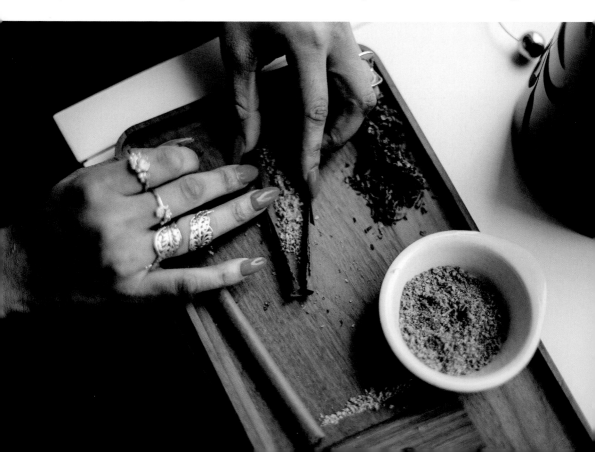

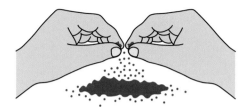

Step 1: Grind Your Cannabis

Break down your cannabis into shake using a grinder or your hands. Using a grinder will help maintain an even burn, while using your hands is the more traditional method and is often preferred to help the blunt burn a little more slowly.

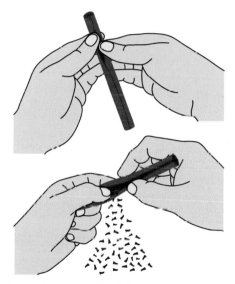

Step 2: Prep the Blunt Wrap

To roll your blunt you'll need an empty tobacco wrap. Traditionally, connoisseurs will empty a cigarillo (like Swisher Sweets, Phillies, or Backwoods), but these days you can find empty wraps at most corner stores.

If you're emptying a cigarillo, use a blade to cut the blunt in half lengthwise, or if you've got the right touch you can "crack" the blunt using your fingers. Once you've split the blunt, empty the tobacco from the middle and discard (or if you like to smoke spliffs, save it for later).

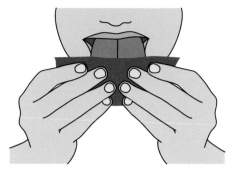

Step 3: Wet the Wrap

Using a small amount of moisture will make your blunt wrap easier to work with and shape, and will help seal up any small tears that might occur while you're emptying its tobacco innards. This is easily done with some saliva, but if you're rolling the blunt for someone else, consider using the tip of your finger and some tap water.

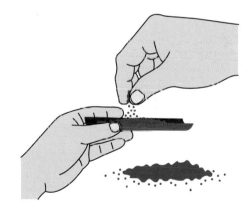

Step 4: Fill It Up

Fill the empty tobacco wrap with ground cannabis. For a standard-size cigarillo one to two grams is plenty, though if you're sharing your blunt, are an experienced roller, or are using a blunt wrap, you should be able to fit a fair amount more.

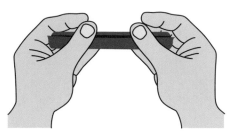

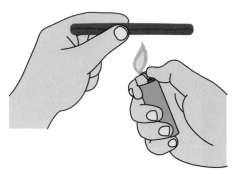

Step 5: Roll the Blunt Wrap

Roll the cannabis between your fingers to pack the blunt evenly. (Be careful: If you didn't moisten the wrap enough, it may crack.) Once you've packed and shaped your blunt, tuck the wrap into itself and wet the inside of the exposed edge from end to end before completing the roll. Use your fingers to smooth out any wrinkles.

> **Leafly Tip:** If you poke a hole or if the blunt cracks at all while you're working with it, you can use the gummy adhesive from rolling papers to repair it.

Step 6: Bake the Blunt

Now that your blunt is rolled, you'll want to "bake" or dry it to help seal it together and encourage an even burn. Bake your blunt by running a lighter lengthwise under the seam and around the outside. Be careful not to hold the lighter too close—you only want the heat, not the flame.

Step 7: Enjoy!

Now that you've got your blunt rolled, all that's left is to light the end and enjoy with some friends!

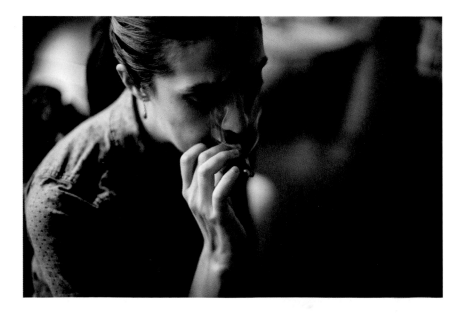

What Is Shake?

LIKE A LOT of cannabis terms, "shake" means different things to different people. And how people define shake does a lot to determine whether they love it or hate it.

"Leftovers" might be the simplest description. Shake consists of small pieces of cannabis flower that break off larger buds, generally as the result of regular shifting or handling. But just like leftovers, shake can be delicious or disgusting. Knowing what to look for in shake can mean the difference between a cool, clean smoke and a coughing fit.

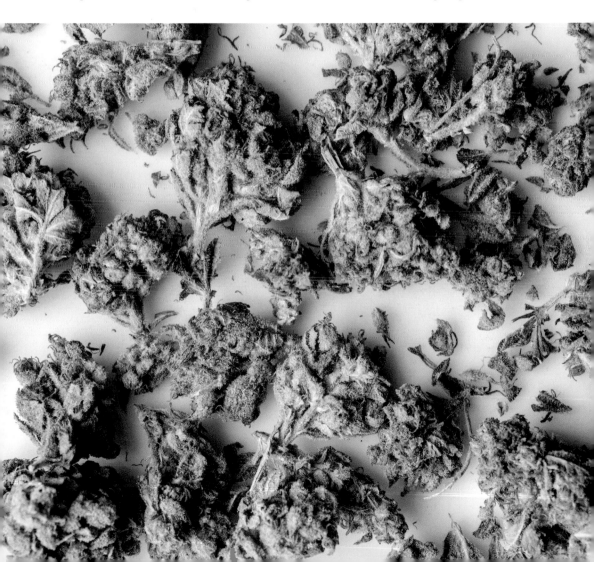

Where to Find It

You're most likely to encounter shake at a medical dispensary, especially one that keeps its flower in large jars. As budtenders shift the nugs, bits break off and collect at the bottom of each jar. The shake is collected and then either sold on its own or used to make pre-rolled joints.

If you buy shake separately, it's almost always cheaper than flower that's still in bud form. So the question becomes whether the discount is worth it. The answer depends largely on what you're looking for in cannabis—and how you plan to consume it. If you're someone who regularly grinds your flower before using it, shake might be worth considering. Joint, blunt, and spliff rollers are an obvious audience, but even fans of glass might be interested if the quality is good and the discount is deep enough. Bakers and other edible makers should also take a look: If you're making cannabutter, it doesn't matter much to have a few small stems and leaves mixed in as long as you'll be straining them out with the rest of the plant matter. You'll also frequently find shake in pre-rolled joints.

Good? Bad? Both?

Does shake deserve its often poor reputation? As it turns out, yes and no.

By definition, shake is just smaller pieces of flower. If the nugs are of good quality, it's reasonable to expect the shake that falls off to be good, too. But that's not always the case. There are a few common reasons why shake gets a bad rap. First, shake can be dry. Usually this is the result of jars being left out too long, but sometimes it's simply because the shake itself is old. With more surface area than tightly packed buds, shake oxidizes much faster (so if you do pick some up, be sure to store it properly).

Another problem with shake is that it can contain stems and other bits of unwanted plant matter—the result of picking apart bigger nugs. Sometimes dispensaries or pre-roll producers will spread shake over screens and remove all that junk, but other times they don't.

Worse still is when growers try to pass off trim as shake. People sometimes use the words interchangeably, but trim is not shake, and shake isn't trim. Trim is the unwanted plant matter that's cut away from cannabis buds before curing. It's not a pleasant smoke—it can smell like a campfire and taste "plant-y"—and it's far less potent than actual shake.

Another consideration for medical patients: Sometimes shake is combined from various strains, so it's important to be clear on what you're getting. Ask questions and explain your needs to dispensary staff. If strain-specific effects are important for your treatment, you may want to avoid so-called mystery or rainbow rolls: pre-rolled joints made from a mix of different strains.

Ultimately, however, shake shouldn't suggest low-quality cannabis any more than leftovers should suggest low-quality food. In certain circumstances, such as rolling joints or making edibles, shake can be a perfect choice, increasing convenience and cutting cost. Like many cannabis products, it's simply a matter of knowing what questions to ask.

Extra Credit: The Doritos Principle

One theory we have on the issue of shake goes like this: Just as the bottom of a bag of Doritos contains smaller, uglier, but incredibly flavorful chip bits, shake should be smaller, uglier, more powerful pieces of cannabis. Right? You're familiar with how Doritos flavor dust works. Isn't shake just little bits of flower rolling around in bottom-of-the-bag kief, the potent gold dust that coats cannabis buds?

Not everyone we talked to saw it that way. But some did. "I wouldn't go so far as to call it more potent," said Corey Schwartz, manager of Los Angeles dispensary Coast to Coast Collective. "I would call them the same." We explained the Doritos Principle, but he pushed back: "It's still the same Doritos." Patrick Rooney at Vashon Velvet, on the other hand, thought there might be something to the idea. "Totally," he said. "That could definitely happen. I've had some bags that are just kief at the bottom. It might be nice to smoke." He even went so far as to say the remnants might have an "excellent cannabinoid profile," but then added, "I just don't think it's consistent enough to market as a product."

Besides, Rooney said, that much kief would take time to accumulate, and time dries out cannabis. "The stuff on the bottom might be potent," he said, "but it's going to really burn your throat."

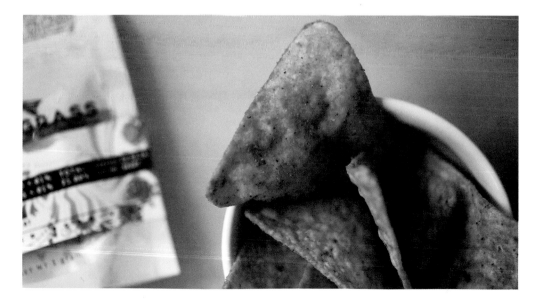

What's in a Pre-Rolled Joint?

MORE THAN PIPES, bongs, edibles, oils, dab rigs, or any other means of consumption, the joint remains an icon. It may be the only consumption method that, when pantomimed, says to the rest of the world, "Hey, that's cannabis!"

A joint is cheap, discreet, disposable, and easily shared among friends. It requires neither the financial investment of a bong nor the time commitment of an edible. But unless you've got nimble fingers or hours to spend practicing, it can be tough to learn how to twist one up.

Enter the pre-roll. Before legal, regulated cannabis markets, consumers themselves were the ones rolling joints. But as medical dispensaries and recreational shops emerged, demand grew for ready-made smokeables. By now, pre-rolls are common, serving as go-to gifts and common suggestions for cannabis newcomers.

There's just one thing: A lot of people think they're junk. But where did that reputation come from? Is it deserved? And does it really mean pre-rolls aren't worth it? A lot of people who disparage pre-rolled joints will, when pressed, admit that they don't actually smoke pre-rolls themselves. So we spoke to budtenders, producers, dispensary owners, and cannabis enthusiasts to set the record straight.

The biggest takeaway? When it comes to pre-rolls, it's hard to generalize. But at least in some markets, they don't always deserve the bad rap. The quality of pre-rolls can vary widely; while some producers use higher-quality flower, others add what's called trim—the leaves and stems that are cut away from the bud before curing. Overall, the biggest problem with a pre-roll is the paper, because it hides what's inside. That makes it easier for unscrupulous producers to get away with using subpar cannabis or trim. Even when a producer uses high-quality cannabis, consumers still can't easily tell what's inside at a glance—so a store may see little advantage in stocking high-quality pre-rolls.

Shake: The Secret Ingredient in Pre-Rolls

Here's how most pre-rolls are made: As budtenders in dispensaries shift nugs of cannabis in their jars, smaller bits of shake (see previous chapter for description) fall off. "The jars get shifted all the time," explained Corey Schwartz, who manages Coast to Coast Collective in Los Angeles. "As you're dispensing to patients, they want certain buds. After a day or half a day, that strain gets broken down." The shake gets collected for use in pre-rolls, which in Coast to Coast's case are rolled on site.

Some producers also add nugs to their pre-roll mixture. From there the mix is loaded into pre-rolled paper cones. A machine shakes the joints to help settle the mixture and remove air pockets. Once the joints are filled, an employee gently tamps down the contents of each one to make sure it's not too tight or too loose, which could cause it to burn poorly. With a twist of the tip, the pre-roll's ready to go.

Including shake in pre-rolls is a widespread practice, and it ensures that all of a dispensary's flower is put to use. But it can also ruffle feathers. Some consumers think shake is low-quality cannabis, which isn't necessarily the case. In essence, shake is just smaller pieces of the same quality stuff.

But there are caveats. Shake can be of low quality if it's dry—usually the result of jars sitting out too long—or if it contains stems and bits of leaves. And sometimes shake from various strains can be combined when making pre-rolls (often called "mystery" or "rainbow" rolls). There's also a bigger problem: Trim masquerading as shake. Before buying a bunch of pre-rolls from a producer or dispensary, it's not a bad idea to sacrifice one and cut it open to see what's inside. The contents should look about the same as if you'd ground up a new nug. It's also okay to just ask your dispensary—in fact, you should.

Pre-Rolls Vary by Market

In Washington, state law requires that all nugs be prepackaged for consumers, so there is no dispensary shake to work with. As such, producers make their own pre-rolls. Vashon Velvet, for instance, uses the same nugs it packages and sells—for the most part. The Vashon Island–based farm packages the prettiest ones from the tops of the plants for consumers, then harvests lower buds to grind and roll into joints. "They're still good-quality cannabis, but they're not quite what we'd want to put in a bag to represent our stuff," said Vashon Velvet's Patrick Rooney. The nugs are ground to a fine consistency and then screened to remove twigs and stems. Once made, the joints are individually inspected and packaged in boxes, then heat-sealed to help keep the cannabis fresh—an important step, according to Rooney.

"I would totally compare it to coffee," he explained. "In the bean form, it's going to last longer than if you grind it. It's going to be a completely different coffee when it's ground." With more surface area in the ground-up cannabis, it will dry out and oxidize faster, leaving you with a harsher, less-potent smoke.

If in doubt, you can always check out the Products section on the Leafly website to find out the best pre-rolls near you.

Tips for Finding Great Pre-Rolls

- Ask your friends for their local favorites.

- Ask your budtender to recommend the freshest products they carry.

- Cut open a pre-roll and compare the look, smell, and feel of what's inside to freshly ground flower.

- Pay attention when you smoke because if producers are adding trim to the mix, quality will be significantly compromised; the joint will smell like a campfire and taste "plant-y."

What's the Deal with Hash?

Extracting kief is one of the first steps of making hash. Hash is basically just kief that has been heated and pressurized to form a soft, green ball. Applying heat and pressure to kief changes its composition by rupturing the resin glands. Once the kief has ruptured, the overall taste and effects of the product are slightly different. Pressurizing kief also darkens its color; the more pressure you apply, the darker the hash becomes.

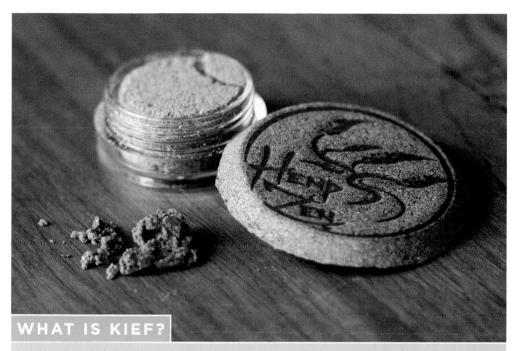

WHAT IS KIEF?

Simply put, kief (also known as dry sift or pollen) refers to the resin glands of the cannabis plant, which contain the terpenes and cannabinoids that make cannabis unique. While marijuana sans kief still contains cannabinoids, the resin glands that develop on flower buds pack the biggest punch. Kief specifically refers to the bulbous, crystal formation on the tip of a gland; that said, the substance itself is just one part of what is called a trichome, or a "hair."

What purpose does kief, and trichomes more generally, serve? It's all about protection. Many different plants and algae have external trichomes for specific evolutionary purposes. Some carnivorous plants rely on sticky trichomes to trap their prey. Trichomes on the cannabis plant keep away hungry herbivores by producing an intense psychoactive experience, theoretically disorienting the animal and preventing it from eating the rest of the plant. The resin's strong, distinct odor also attracts pollinating insects and predators, which might keep herbivore populations at bay.

What is kief used for? Everything from making hash to sprinkling over bowls and into joints to increase potency. Kief may not be the most exciting cannabis product out there, but it still remains one of the most popular and easiest to access.

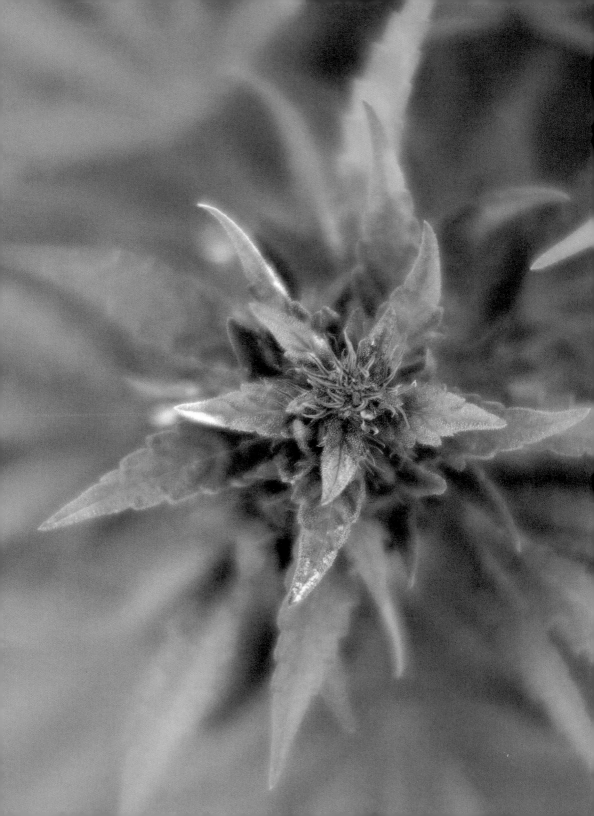

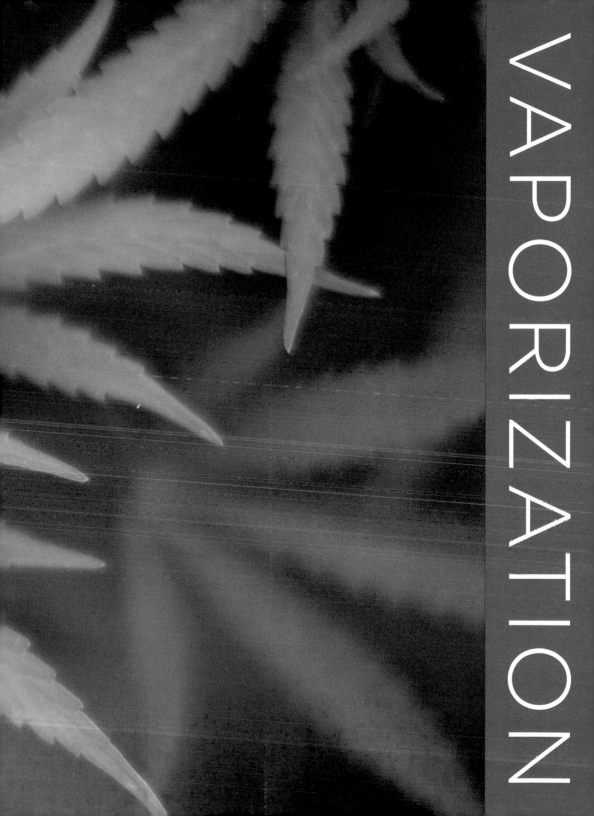

VAPORIZATION

How Does Vaporization Work?

VAPORIZATION IS THE process whereby cannabis flowers or concentrates are heated to a temperature that releases cannabinoids and terpenoids to create an inhalable vapor, but does not induce combustion, or burning. Vaporizing is healthier than smoking, and also produces near-instant effects. With ever more compact and technologically advanced vaporizer models on the market, vaporization continues to grow steadily in popularity.

Many consumers are attracted to vapor for a simple reason: Researchers feel it's one of the healthiest consumption methods. Combusting cannabis creates toxins—including some carcinogens— that disturb the respiratory system;

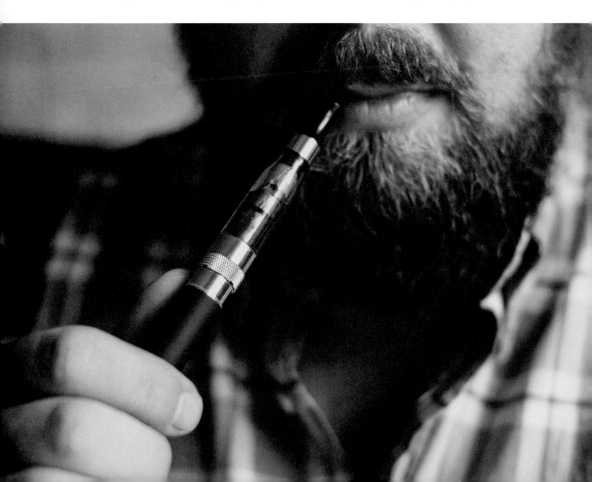

vaporization, on the other hand, is a smokeless method that heats cannabis at a much lower temperature, releasing cannabinoids and terpenes into a vapor without the harmful by-products. Vaporizers may work with dried cannabis flower, cannabis concentrates, or both.

Another benefit of vaporization lies in its ability to preserve unique flavors and nuanced effects in cannabis flowers and concentrates. Much in the same way that fine wine displays elements of *terroir*, cannabis, too, can vary based on where and how it was grown. Whereas combustion burns off many of the naturally occurring components that govern variation in cannabis aromas, flavors, and psychotropic effects, vaporization preserves these elements. As such, many who consider themselves cannabis connoisseurs prefer this method of ingestion over others.

Conduction vs. Convection

Different components of the cannabis plant vaporize at different temperatures. Certain cannabinoids begin to vaporize around 284°F; by contrast, combustion doesn't begin until around 446°F. Vaporizers apply heat between those two temperatures. They do so using one of two types of heating mechanisms that extract active ingredients from plant matter, converting them to vapor. Some vapes even allow consumers to control the temperature, thus controlling the cannabinoids and terpenes that are released and consumed.

Conductive Heating

In conductive vaporizers, dried flower or extracts are placed directly onto an electronically heated surface, most often a solid metal or a screen. The "hot plate" is then heated to an ideal vaporization temperature, directing heat throughout the chamber and converting the cannabinoids and terpenes into vapor.

Convective Heating

With convection heating, the cannabis product doesn't come in contact with the heating element. Once the air has reached the ideal temperature, it is moved by either a fan or inhalation to the component containing the cannabis product, heating the flower or concentrate and converting the cannabinoids and terpenes into vapor without charring the substance. Convection heating elements are generally made with ceramic, though some use stainless steel.

What to Consider When Choosing a Vaporizer

IF YOU'RE THINKING of purchasing a vaporizer, there are four important things to keep in mind.*

Flower vs. Concentrate

This is probably the number-one question you'll want to ask yourself: "Do I want to refill with cannabis flower or concentrate?" If you enjoy smoking and are planning on splitting time between your vaporizer and, say, rolling papers, you will probably want a vaporizer that takes loose-leaf so you don't have to purchase both flower and concentrates. If you are planning on ditching smoking for vaporizing (perhaps due to health concerns

*As with all apparatus, check legality before purchasing.

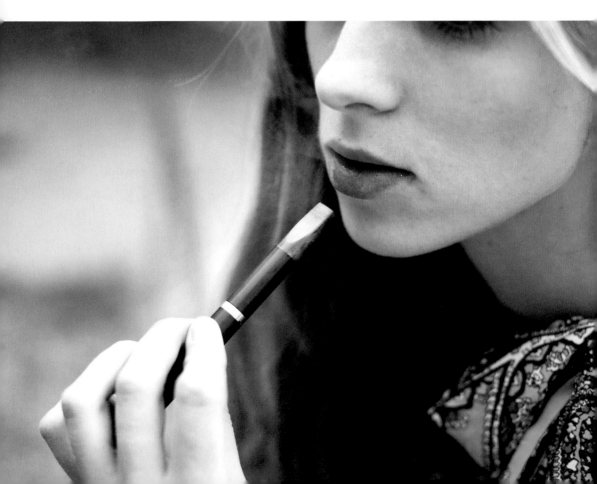

associated with smoking), you can commit full-time to concentrates unabashedly. That said, many people prefer the flexibility of a vaporizer that can handle both.

From an economic standpoint, flower and concentrate vaporizers are different beasts. Concentrate cartridges run at about forty dollars a pop and provide anywhere from a hundred to two hundred pulls from the pen, whereas flower vapes operate by the traditional "bowl" system: The chamber is comparable to an average-size bowl, with the cost of filling dependent upon the cannabis strain, quality, provider, and so on.

Keep in mind that in terms of strain selection, in today's market, flowers offer a much greater variety than concentrates. So if you're a connoisseur of sorts, a loose-leaf vaporizer will still provide you with plenty of room for exploration. However, market growth is expected to be vast and fast for concentrates, so the future is bright for fans of oils, shatters, rosins, and waxes.

Efficiency

Didn't think you'd ever need to recall the difference between conduction and convection, did you? Turns out Chem 101 was useful for, if nothing else, making an informed loose-leaf vaporizer purchase. Conduction and convection describe heat transfer: Conduction is motionless (think metal against plant material), whereas convection requires liquid or gas to move the energy (think steam).

Convective vaporizers are—in theory—more efficient; conductive heating is often uneven (flower touching the chamber walls will receive more heat than flower in the center of the chamber) and inefficient (they heat continuously, even when you aren't inhaling, which can waste flower). Depending on how tightly you pack a conduction vape chamber, you may also have to stir the flower after a couple pulls to achieve even heating. That said, this point is moot if you're going with concentrates, where the need to decarboxylate (activate) the cannabinoids has been eliminated.

Convenience

This comes down to how you want to use your vaporizer. If it's a quick, on-the-go, one-two puff you prefer, concentrates make a lot of sense: There is no heating time, and vape pens are usually small and inconspicuous. Alternatively, if you're looking to hold group sessions or only vape at home, a loose-leaf flower vape that requires some heating time is less of an issue.

Preparing the device is an important consideration: For loose-leaf vaporizers, the chamber must be loaded before every use with ground flower (don't forget your grinder), and the vape should be cleaned regularly. Concentrates can go either way: Some take screw-in, disposable cartridges while others require loading. The process of loading concentrates can get messy if you don't have the right tools, but luckily concentrate refills are needed much less frequently.

Battery life and recharge time are also important considerations; battery-run loose-leaf vaporizers have an on-off switch and continuously drain power while they're on, with a charge life comparable to a laptop. Alternatively, most vape pens do not have an on-off switch and only use power when you are vaping, reducing the frequency of recharging.

Along those same lines, if portability isn't a factor, an entire subset of plug-in, stationary vaporizers become viable options.

Experience

If the experience of smoking is a great joy for you, you have a vested interest in experiencing the taste and smell of the plant. Trial and error is the best method for finding the vape that suits your palate, but in general, loose-leaf vapes provide a stronger taste than concentrates. Furthermore, the smell of flower that has already been vaped is potent and often objectionable (think burnt toast), meaning you'll want to empty your loose-leaf chamber shortly after each use, which is not a concern for concentrates.

Lastly, many people covet the headiness that comes with smoking. Vaping usually produces lighter effects. This can be good or bad depending on what you're looking for—for some this means *clearer* effects; for others it means *weaker* effects.

Pens vs. Portables vs. Tabletop Vaporizers

What's the Difference?

LIVING IN A tech-forward era comes with many conveniences, but also with "burdens"—such as choosing a vaporizer in an endless sea of options. A changing legal climate has given rise to all kinds of newfangled vaping contraptions that deliver your desired effects with unprecedented precision, efficiency, safety, and quality of flavor. How to choose the best one?

First and foremost, it's a good idea to familiarize yourself with some of the basics before diving into further research on specific brands.*

*Check the legality applicable to you before purchasing.

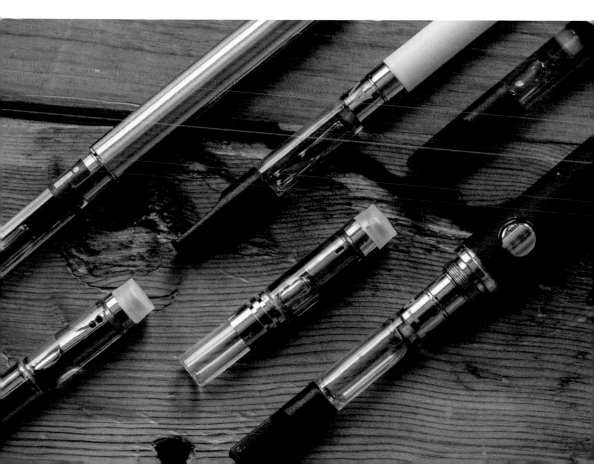

Tabletop Vaporizers

Refers to: Larger vaporizers that plug into a power source.

Ideal for: Homebodies, flavor enthusiasts, medical patients.

Portability: If you're the type of person who only indulges at home, your best option is likely a tabletop vaporizer. Due to their size and dependence on a wall outlet, this vaporizer probably won't leave your house often, if at all. They generally come with a hoselike mouthpiece or a bag that fills with the vapor so you can inhale at your own pace. These stationary vapes aren't ideal for the one-hit-and-done type of person, but they're excellent options for sharing and for those who'd normally conquer a full bowl by themselves.

Functionality: Though often too clunky to conveniently lug around, these setups tend to offer the most advanced technology among vaporizers. But, of course, it depends on how much you're willing to invest. Some of the better devices can cost several hundred dollars, but offer precise and adjustable temperature control. This is important as different cannabinoids and terpenes— all with their own unique effects and medical benefits—vaporize at different temperatures. Also, if you're a fiend for good flavor, a nice tabletop vaporizer will go a long way. Cheaper ones can make your bud taste like burnt popcorn, but high-quality devices tend to deliver vapor that stays true to the flower's natural aroma.

Quality of Effects: Precise temperature controls allow you to target specific cannabinoids and terpenes, so the effect profile may change depending on which ones you're aiming for. For example, the terpene pinene usually helps with alertness and memory and vaporizes at 311°F. You can play around with temperature to see how it changes your experience!

Portable Flower Vapes

Refers to: Smaller, battery-powered vaporizers with a chamber for cannabis flower.

Ideal for: On-the-go flower enthusiasts.

Portability: Generally speaking, portability is about the only reason you'd invest in a portable flower vape over a stationary tabletop device. Because they're small and run on a battery, these vaporizers don't restrict you to one spot at home. They also tend to be cheaper than tabletop vapes, with high-quality products costing around two to three hundred dollars.

Functionality: While these vaporizers have the advantage of portability, their functionality is often more limited. Many flower vaporizers heat the flower at a single fixed temperature, which may be too hot if you're trying to get more of those flavorful terpenes. Some permit you to manipulate the heat but may not allow you to choose a specific temperature. However, flower vapes allow you to choose and consume specific strains, whereas strain-specific cartridges and concentrates for oil pens are rarer—often, concentrates are derived from blends of many different strains.

Portable Oil Vapes

Refers to: Small, battery-powered vaporizers that use oil instead of flower.

Ideal for: On-the-go concentrate enthusiasts, small budgets.

Portability: Preferred for their portability and discretion, portable oil vapes are perfect for the mobile oil enthusiast. Some don't require loading or unloading product—it all comes neatly contained in a sealed cylindrical oil cartridge, which screws directly onto the battery of your pen. Others, however, can be filled with your own cannabis oil.

Functionality: Vaporizers that look just like a pen or a stylus are gaining popularity because the batteries are inexpensive and the CO2 oil inside them hits smoothly and lasts a long time. Some have had issues with battery life and leakage, but these are generally rare malfunctions. Vaporizers that require you to load your own oils can be great alternatives for those without access to cartridges, but sometimes getting the right consistency of oil can be tricky.

Quality of Effects: Although portable vapes don't often give you the temperature control found in tabletop devices, they can still capture some of the nuances of each unique strain. Portable vaporizers with some level of temperature customization are often preferred to those without, as they can be turned down if the product tastes burnt or turned up if you aren't getting a full enough vapor.

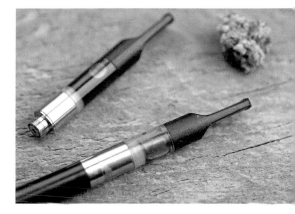

Quality of Effects: You may notice that the CO2 oil in cartridge pens offers distinctly different effects from other types of cannabis oil. For some, the high is often more cerebrally focused with fewer body effects, although these sensations vary across brands and strains. Cartridge oils are often diluted with propylene glycol (also used in e-cigarettes), a solvent used to achieve the right consistency for vaping. These solvents are not a concern for noncartridge vaporizers; it's up to you which oil you decide to put in these.

The Volcano

A Brief History of the World's Most Iconic Vaporizer

THE HISTORY OF vaporization is unfolding in front of us, and if a single product were to be named as founder of the vaporization industry, it would be the Volcano by Storz & Bickel. This stylish tabletop vaporizer practically invented the market for modern alternatives to combustion and has since gone on to experience great success and acclaim. Volcano vaporizers have embodied the gold standard in vaporization technology since their arrival in European and American markets in the late '90s and early 2000s. But before they were expanding across the oceans or sponsoring Cannabis Cups, Storz & Bickel were just a pair of gentlemen in pursuit of a higher and healthier standard for enjoying cannabis.

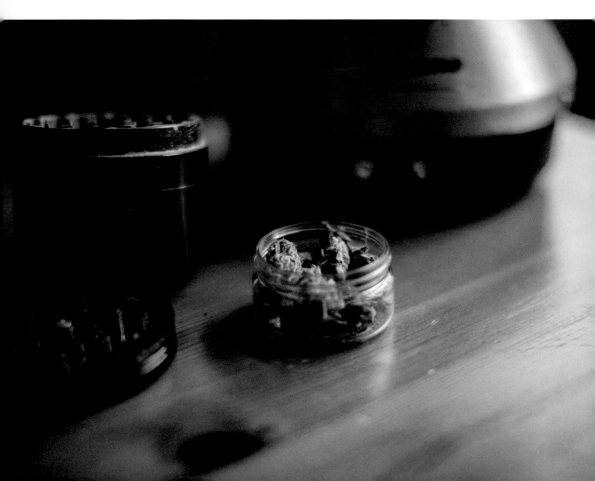

Markus Storz began his career as a "qualified graphic designer." His artistic education would be a natural complement to his partner's technical background, but that is not to say Storz didn't possess a great deal of ingenuity himself. Unable to find a suitable herbal vaporizer that met his standards, Storz began development on the Volcano in 1996. As with many acts in the company's narrative, the Volcano would arise out of a search for quality, consistency, and the highest standards possible.

Early Product Experimentation

The first iteration of the Volcano was created in Storz's cellar using a Steinel heat gun. Though this process would prove unsatisfactory due to carbon residue, it was a necessary first step toward the innovation of the air pump found in the modern Volcano vaporizer. The use of forced air was in response to the popularity of "bulb" (or "whip") vaporizers, whose steady flow of heated air dispersed more evenly amid plant matter, ensuring a more efficient use of the herbal materials. Volcano patented a detachable balloon chamber for its vaporizer in 1998, which proved to be the jewel in the company's crown.

The balloon was specifically designed to separate the vaporization and inhalation processes, keeping the patient out of contact with the vaporizer and the heat created by vaporization. Also, the balloon system allowed for a second party (a nurse or caretaker) to prepare a patient's inhalation dose, and the balloon itself has little to no resistance on the inhale, making it perfect for the ill or disabled. The consistent and reproducible nature of the Volcano balloon made it an ideal delivery method for medicinal use and study.

Jürgen Bickel, a longtime friend of Storz, acquired his first Volcano in the same cellar where it had been invented. Bickel was a German civil engineer working in Peru, who specialized in potable water supply and treatment. Bickel preferred vaporization to smoking the local hash cigarettes, and managed to bring along Storz's invention for personal use over his five-year stay in the Andes. Having found kindred spirits in each other, the two entrepreneurs made the partnership official in 2002, and Storz & Bickel was born.

Bickel says attaining funding, patents, and industry certifications were arduous facets of forming the company, but necessary pillars of the business, especially with their sights set on the medical industry. The medical market compounded the company's relationship to medicinal cannabis, but also necessitated a standard of quality that Storz and Bickel admired. In 2003 their hard work paid off when the company was awarded the Dr. Rudolf Eberle Prize for outstanding technical innovation.

From Innovators to Industry Leaders

With cannabis gaining popularity around the globe and innovation as the company's mandate, Storz & Bickel released the Volcano Digit in 2007. This allowed for more accurate temperature control designed to help pinpoint temperatures at which certain terpenes and cannabinoids vaporized, expanding the vaporizer's applications to the culinary and concentrate markets. This wave of innovation would be the first of many over nearly a decade of ceaseless invention. The Plenty arrived in 2008 and was the first vaporizer to combine air- and radiation-heating methods. This nod to both adult-use and medical cannabis would only further the company's ethos on its way to achieving medical-grade certification in 2009.

The medical-grade materials and quality management systems that Storz & Bickel built into their manufacturing process certified their company and their products as the first ever medical-use vaporizers. This prestigious distinction was something Volcano had been aspiring to since the company's creation. The next six years were dedicated to invention and innovation, giving the cannabis community the Volcano Medic (the world's first medical cannabis inhaler), the Volcano Mighty and Volcano Crafty (mobile, battery powered vaporizers for the masses), and the Volcano Mighty Medic (a battery powered successor of the original Medic).

In the meantime, Volcano grew as a household name and was featured at Cannabis Cups in Amsterdam and abroad. Bickel explained that the company gave several Volcano Vaporizers to cafés in Amsterdam for the Cannabis Cup and each year would send technicians to clean and maintain the vaporizers in conjunction with annual return of the Cup.

Volcano and Storz & Bickel continue to grow and align themselves with the health-oriented imperatives that helped start their company. This year, Volcano is building its Vapor Factory in Tuttlingen, Germany, a town with a reputation for being the nexus of medical technology with nearly five hundred medical device manufacturers located there. With an array of products and no sign of slowing down, Storz & Bickel continue to define the vaporization industry one product at a time.

Vaping Flower vs. Vaping Concentrates

CANNABIS CONCENTRATES ARE becoming an increasingly popular consumption method, but a lot of people new to concentrates feel intimidated by them. This isn't completely unjustified when you consider the learning curve and tolerance adjustment required for concentrates. Because concentrates are a lot more potent than flower and are often associated with complicated consumption technology, why bother switching to something intimidating and confusing when flower seems so much easier and more familiar?

There are several potential benefits to be derived from concentrate consumption, but before you get to vaping, get started with these five basic concentrate facts.

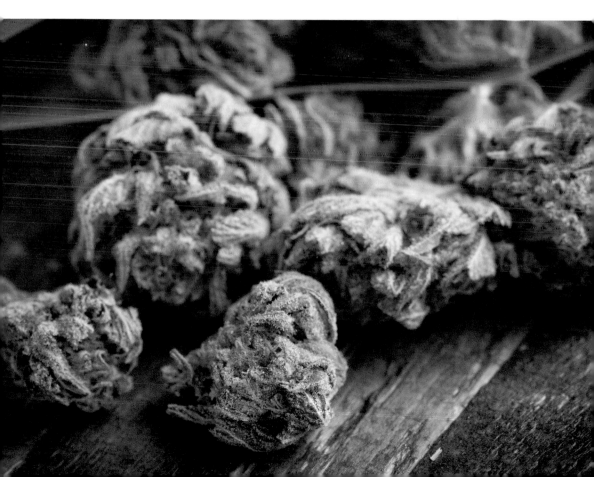

1. Concentrates Go by Many Names

Although the multiplicity of strains available can make one's head spin, even beginners have a pretty good idea of what they're getting with flower, regardless of its name. "Concentrates" is an umbrella term that refers to a variety of different cannabis extracts and their monikers—and that's where things can get more confusing.

Imagine you're standing at the glass counter of a dispensary. Inside you see the following items: shatter, rosin, BHO, CO2, wax, crumble, honey oil, dabs, hash,

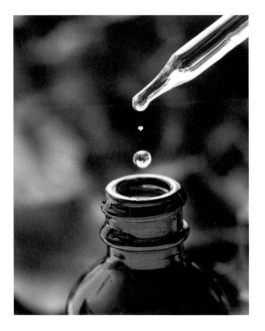

tinctures, and capsules. Don't let the breadth of options drive you away—many of these are different names for the same thing. Here are some quick tips for narrowing your search down:

- Shatter, wax, crumble, sugar, honeycomb, sap, and oil often refer to a concentrate's texture. While some people have a consistency preference, what's important to many people is the solvent used to make the extract and how compatible that extract is with their preferred consumption method.

- Most concentrates are extracted using CO_2, butane, hydrocarbons, propane, water, alcohol, and heat. Solventless extracts made using water (e.g., hash) or heat (e.g., rosin) are excellent choices for those wary of how consuming solvents might affect them.

- Ask your budtender which oils work with your delivery method of choice. Looking to dab something? Consider trying the recommended shatter, hash oil, or CO2 oil. Do you prefer vape pens? Choose a cartridge that's compatible with your battery. Interested in ingestible concentrates? Ask about dosing tinctures and oil capsules.

2. Concentrates Are More Potent

The most important distinction between cannabis flowers and concentrates is potency. While bud potency tends to range between 10 to 25 percent THC, a concentrate typically falls between 50 to 80 percent (and some extracts can even push past 90 percent). Those numbers may be enough to scare off any unseasoned consumers, and for good reason: dosing gets trickier as potency increases.

A mildly or nonpsychoactive CBD-rich concentrate would be a good choice for beginners (that's right, not all concentrates are designed to get you sky high). Hash and tinctures also tend to have lower THC contents than other types of concentrates, so you might consider steering toward those before graduating to the more potent oils. Just remember to always start with a low dose and work your way up if you're new to concentrates or have a low tolerance.

3. Concentrates Can Be Administered Differently

With bud, you can smoke it, vaporize it, and roll it, but there's not much else you can do with it. Concentrates offer more options.

Dabbing: The process by which you apply an extract to a hot nail and inhale the resultant vapor through a glass piece is swiftly on the rise among cannabis enthusiasts. Dabbing is an easy way to get a potent dose of cannabinoids, though the learning curve, safety considerations, and equipment demands make it a less accessible option for new users.

Ingestible oils act like edibles in that they take effect slowly and last much longer due to the way they're metabolized. These oils (or any extract, really) can be high in THC, CBD, or both. So if you're interested in smoke-free methods of consumption—especially for treating medical symptoms and conditions—oil capsules may be worth looking into.

Tinctures are a sublingual concentrate, meaning they're dropped under the tongue and enter the bloodstream from there. They act faster than edibles and ingestible oils, though they're often less potent.

Hash and oils may be consumed using some of the same methods as flower. Some vaporizers are compatible with "loose" oils, though most portable pens are specially designed to be used with specific cartridges. Motivated enthusiasts can even augment their standard bud-packed joints with hash and oils for added potency.

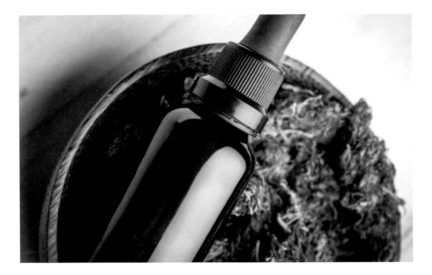

4. Plant Matter Is Stripped from Concentrates

When you smoke flower, you're also smoking the plant material that leaves your glass black with tar. That can take a toll on your lungs. However, you may have noticed that when you dab oils, the glass and water stay clean for much longer. In concentrates, extraction processes strip out plant material and isolate the compounds you want like THC and CBD, which is a major benefit for many consumers. That said, some things you don't want, like pesticides, contaminants, and residual solvents, can also be concentrated in oils, shatters, and waxes; make sure the products you consume are tested for contaminants prior to consuming them.

5. Flowers May Have More Flavor and Terpenes, but Not Always

If flavor is something you care about, be aware that some concentrates will lose their aromas and flavors in the extraction process. Terpenes are the volatile, fragrant oils secreted by the cannabis plant, and they give the flowers their smells from the sweet, fruity, and floral to the earthy, piney, and musky. Being sensitive to heat, terpenes are difficult to preserve in many extraction processes.

For this reason, many producers have begun reintroducing these aromatic compounds afterward—which can result in products even more flavorful than the flower they came from.

An Experiment

BY LEAFLY EDITOR, BAILEY RAHN

Many cannabis consumers think customizing their cannabis buzz is limited to the strains on the shelves, but temperature is an equally important factor that impacts your experience. Think of temperature control as the key to unlocking the full array of effects a strain can offer. A strain that's high in CBD (nonpsychoactive, relaxing, antiepileptic), for example, must be heated to the compound's boiling point of 356°F if you're to reap its benefits. Likewise, the relaxing terpene linalool isn't unleashed until you hit 388°F. Temperature can also determine a strain's intensity: higher temperatures typically exaggerate effects, while lower temperatures offer a gentler, more mellow experience.

This type of customization isn't possible through smoking. When you bring a lighter to your bowl, you're combusting the plant material, which creates smoke, carbon dioxide, and other harmful by-products. The temperature is hot enough to activate the THC and other compounds, but this "sledgehammer approach" isn't terribly efficient, as temperatures that high can also destroy volatile but pertinent cannabinoids and terpenes.

Knowing that cannabis has a variety of precious constituents with different boiling points, I wanted to see how temperature affected the overall experience felt by different strains. Lining up a row of strain jars like test tubes, I turned on my trusty tabletop vaporizer and began playing mad scientist.

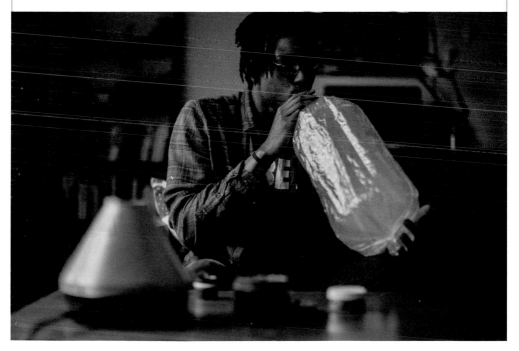

LOW TEMPERATURES FOR CLEARHEADED, FUNCTIONAL EFFECTS

310°F to 330°F
Possible effects: mild euphoria, focus, productivity, subtle relaxation

There's a time and place to be stoned off your rocker, but sometimes all you need is the slightest kick from your cannabis. For days when you need uplifting relief to carry you through chores and tasks, low-temp vaping is the key to a functional, productive buzz.

I loaded my Headband concentrate and set my vaporizer to 320°F in order to release three key constituents: the uplifting, focus-feeding terpene pinene; the pepper-flavored anti-inflammatory terpene caryophyllene; and of course, the psychoactive commander in chief, THC. Despite high levels of THC, vaporizing at this temperature didn't make me feel stoned in the slightest. Instead, I was left feeling acutely alert and in complete control of my faculties. The taste was a subtle mix of herbs and pine, but certainly lacked the loud flavors found at higher temperatures.

Turning the heat up to 330°F, the high became slightly more intense but tasks and concentration were still completely manageable. The 290°F to 330°F range seems the perfect fit for those who wish to stay productive and functional, cannabis novices and newbies, and/or anyone sensitive to THC's side effects (dizziness, paranoia, dry eyes/mouth, lethargy, et cetera).

MODERATE TEMPERATURES FOR A BALANCED BUZZ

330°F to 370°F
Possible effects: moderate euphoria, enhanced sensory awareness, mood elevation, functional relaxation

As you increase the heat, more THC is volatilized and your high becomes more intense. This middle range—330°F to 370°F—gives rise to more euphoric effects that help elevate the mood, stimulate giggles, and kick-start the appetite. It's more functional than when you push past the 370°F mark, but you will most definitely start to feel the high that lower temperatures spared you.

Historically, 365°F has been the sweet spot for me (I'll never forget because the first time I vaporized, my friend read the machine's clock-like screen and thought it was 3:65 p.m.). I've always loved the combination of tamed euphoria coupled with the subtle relaxation and focus found at this temperature. I turned my vape up to 365°F and dished out more of the Headband wax. The vapor felt fuller than it did at 330°F, and the flavor was perfectly fruity with the aftertaste of sweet vanilla and licorice. Its effects were distinctly different from the low-temp experience: my thoughts went from a sloppy sprint to a relaxed walking pace, allowing me to unwind and focus.

Whether you're kicking back with a book, exercising, socializing, cleaning, or playing video games, these moderate temperatures provide most of the cannabinoids and terpenes you want without fully volatilizing the THC—I know many people who want as much THC as possible, but for others it's about achieving a careful balance of clearheadedness and blissful elevation.

HIGH TEMPERATURES FOR INTENSE EUPHORIA AND RELAXATION

370°F to 430°F

Possible effects: Intense euphoria, sleep, heavy relaxation, meditation

For ultimate THC decarboxylation mode, turn your vaporizer above 370°F. At these high temperatures, you get terpenes like linalool (calming, anxiety relieving) and cannabinoids like THCV (energizing, appetite suppressing), but keep in mind that they're approaching combustion territory. You may even notice the vapor becomes smokier and harsher on the lungs.

Durban Poison is a South African sativa known for its elevated levels of THCV, a highly psychoactive cannabinoid known to weaken appetite (yes, weaken). I coincidentally had this strain in my collection last week, so I decided to cook it at 430°F to see if I felt more energized than I would at a lower temperature.

For me, the answer was a definitive yes. I started inhaling the bag of Durban Poison fumes (a little bit went a long way) and shared it with my roommate when I realized how high I had become after just a few hits. I passed the kitchen on my way out, and caught a glance of those old-fashioned glazed chocolate doughnuts—the kind you'd normally eat like popcorn after getting stoned. Call it a THCV placebo or miracle, but those seductive delicacies had no power over me (until later, but that's irrelevant).

Vaporizing the indica Skywalker at a high temperature—390°F to be specific—was an entirely different story. My muscles melted, eyelids got heavy, and thoughts became shrouded in a pleasant mental mist that made it easy to fall into a calm, meditative state. I can't say for certain whether it's the linalool gained at 388°F or the more fully volatilized THC, but this strain was detectably heavier at higher temperatures and decidedly more sedating than the Durban Poison when vaporized at the same temperature. That brings us to the final and most obvious consideration when attempting to customize an experience: the strain.

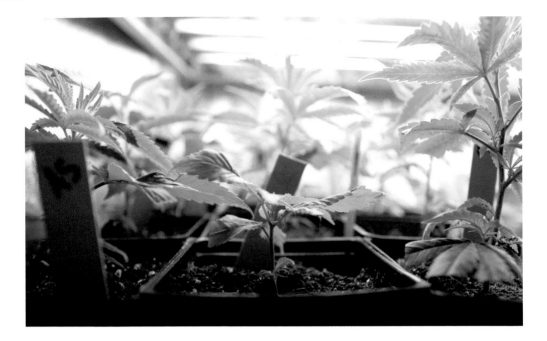

Temperature Variation vs. Strain Variation

The aforementioned temperature tiers don't so much "create" effects—they modify them, so keep in mind that the limits of your customization are set by whatever strain you're working with. Take Durban Poison and Skywalker as examples. Between a racy, upbeat sativa and a heavy, pacifying indica, Durban Poison will always have that high-energy cerebral-effect profile and Skywalker is destined to be a calming sedative (in most people's opinions). Temperature is basically the volume knob: turn it up for intensity, and turn it down for subtlety.

In summary, don't forget that with increases in temperature, you can uncork more essential compounds; however, go too hot and you may be destroying some of those delicate cannabinoids and terpenes. Everyone has their own preference, and it's up to you to find your own favorite temperature, but knowing exactly what is vaporizing at those temperatures may help.

Vaping vs. Dabbing

Why You Should Care About Heat

■ WALK AROUND ANY hemp festival or Cannabis Cup in the United States and you'll notice two products all over the place: vaporizers and dab rigs. In many ways, these trends represent two competing directions for the cannabis industry.

On one hand, vaporization has blown up as a health trend for cannabis lovers. Most forms of cannabis consumption have some type of downside: Smoking cannabis, for instance, still subjects the consumer to charred plant matter, and many edible companies still rely on sugary desserts as a vehicle for infused products. Vaporizing your cannabis is the only surefire way to avoid the most common cons to cannabis consumption, since the process doesn't create smoke and is 100 percent calorie- and sugar-free.

On the other hand (and much to the horror of the typical cannabis naysayer), dabbing has also risen dramatically in popularity. Yet the biggest opposition to dabbing doesn't have as much to do with health as the general appearance of the activity—when you take a blowtorch to a metal nail, consuming marijuana suddenly looks almost entirely like consuming something else (not to mention the obvious safety considerations of operating a blowtorch).

To better understand the role that heating technologies play in your cannabis consumption, here's a quick lesson in their basic mechanics, including expert insight from Seibo Shen of VapeXhale.

Vaporization vs. Dabbing (Or Conductive vs. Convective Heating)

In many ways, dabbing is actually healthier than smoking. Yet for enthusiasts trying to consume cannabis in the safest way possible, there are a few things to understand about what's happening to the cannabis when it's heated in particular ways. Vaporizers and other tools that rely on conduction to transform cannabis product into smoke or vapor typically use flower or concentrate directly applied to a hot plate to change a product into a useable form. When dabbing, the "hot plate" is an ultra-hot nail that is heated to extremely high temperatures using a small blowtorch (and that amount of heat requires caution—enthusiasts should be careful when dabbing).

"Dabbing may be less harmful than smoking," explained Shen, "but it's still not vaporizing. When you're heating the nail 900 to 1,000 degrees and you're dropping some oils onto it and watching it sizzle, that pad is getting hotter than a frying pan when you're frying your food. Those char marks that are created, that's combustion."

Rather than heating the cannabis matter directly with a heating element, convective vaporization uses an electronic mechanism to heat air. Once the air reaches a certain temperature, the hot air heats the cannabis flower or concentrate in turn, extracting the THC and turning the material into a vapor without charring the substance. Of the two types, convective vaporization creates the purest form of activated, consumable cannabis, and is the best for your body.

It's What's Inside That Counts

Though vaporization is one of the healthiest ways to consume cannabis, not all vaporizers are created equal. Depending on the model, some vaporizers rely on the same methods for activating and extracting cannabinoids as other consumption methods, like dabbing. As the vaporizer market grows, consumers need to understand what to look for in a quality machine.

"When we began looking at vape after vape, we noticed a common trend: the heater is sitting in the same chamber as the electronics," said Shen. "As in many electrical devices, most of the individual components are held together by solder. This is concerning because when that heating element begins to warm up the solder, that metal can begin off gassing. The last thing someone who is conscious of their health wants to be concerned about is inhaling anything other than cannabis vapor."

Not only that, but vaporizers that rely on adding water to the machine may face an additional problem: "Many vaporizers use aluminum heaters, which are perfectly fine, but if any sort of moisture happens to get down into the heating chamber, that metal will begin to oxidize and it can rust. Obviously you don't want to inhale something that's rusted."

Too Hot to Handle

The final thing that you need to be concerned about when vaping, dabbing, or relying on heat to consume your herb is temperature. Oftentimes, avid cannabis consumers turn up the heat on their vaporizers (or try to make their dab rigs boiling-lava hot) to produce an extra-thick vapor or smoke. This creates a major problem: benzene.

Benzene is a common carcinogen that can be found in everything from car exhaust to soft drinks to tobacco. While cannabis tends to produce low levels of benzene (a 1986 study found that benzene levels in cannabis consumers are lower than those of tobacco consumers, but higher than nonsmokers), the chemical can still be released when consumers heat their product over 365°F. As such, those vaping for health reasons should stay below that temperature mark.

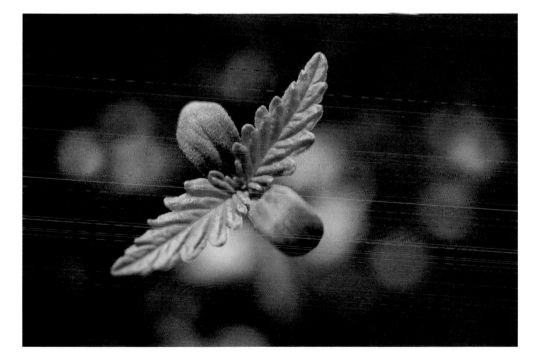

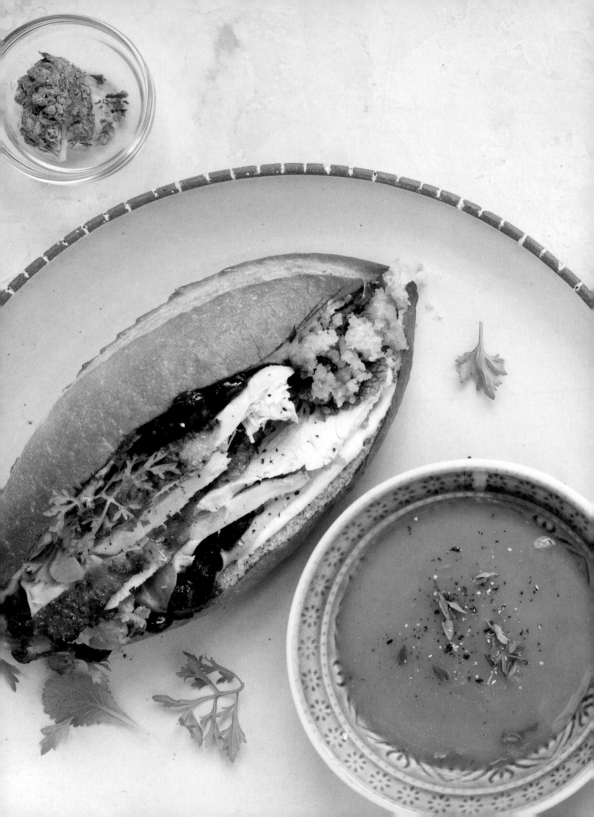

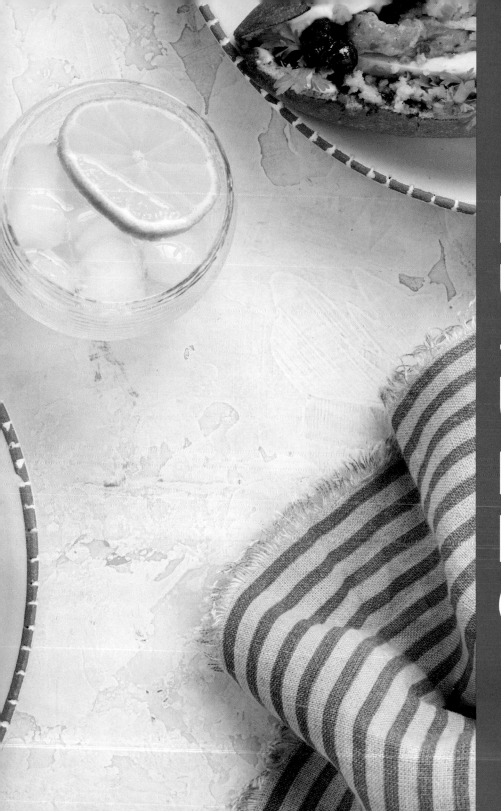

EDIBLES

Edibles 101

EDIBLES ARE HOMEMADE or professionally produced food products that have been infused with cannabis extracts, also known as medibles. Commonly they are baked goods, such as cookies and brownies, but options as varied as salad dressings, savory entrées, and sodas exist as well. When consumed, the activated components of the cannabis plant are absorbed through the digestive system rather than directly into the bloodstream; the resultant high is unique and requires longer to take effect.*

Many of us new to cannabis-infused foods fall victim to the same mistake: We eat too much. Edibles are a great choice for patients when consumed responsibly; they're potent and body-focused, meaning they're perfect for people who suffer from pain, nausea, or lack of appetite.

On the other hand, they can easily lead to disaster if you're not careful. You eat

*The U.S. FDA has not evaluated cannabis products, as cannabis is not legal federally. The legality varies state-by-state, and you should check the laws as applicable to you.

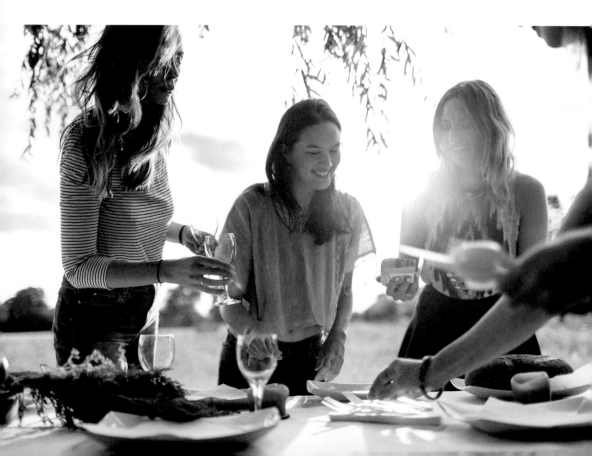

a whole brownie and feel normal for an hour, then all of a sudden you think everyone in the room is secretly laughing at you or start to feel queasy.

In order to help the medi-curious know what to expect from infused foods, Leafly enlisted the help of Lindsay from Dixie Elixirs, one of Colorado's premier edibles manufacturers, to weigh in on some handy tips on how to consume edibles responsibly.

Lesson #1: It Takes Time

When you smoke or vaporize cannabis, you feel the effects of the herb almost instantly. You're also able to see the amount of cannabis you're consuming, which makes it much easier to decide when to stop. When you eat (or drink) activated cannabis, these signals go away, since your body needs to digest and metabolize the food before you feel the effects. That's why the golden rule of edibles is "start low and go slow."

The amount of time it takes for effects to kick in also depends on your metabolism. People with faster metabolisms may observe noticeable effects after an hour, while others with slower metabolisms may have to wait two hours or more. Another important factor is whether you consumed the edible on an empty stomach or after you've already eaten. An empty stomach will help you feel the effects much more quickly, while on a full stomach the effects won't hit you as hard. In order to avoid feeling uncomfortable or sick when eating an infused product, you may want to take Lindsay's advice: "Eat a meal, and then try an edible. Not vice versa. Food doesn't have the same effect for edibles as it does for alcohol. If you feel like you have taken too much, eating a meal can actually push more into your system rather than dilute what's already there."

Lesson #2: Delivery Method Matters

Different delivery systems can mean different rates of absorption into the bloodstream. The THC in infused mints is absorbed in the mouth, and reaches the bloodstream quickly; when THC is contained in fat molecules, as with brownies made using cannabutter, it needs to be processed by the liver before the consumer feels the effects, which slows the process down. The liver will filter out some THC, but it will convert the rest to 11-hydroxy-THC. This active metabolite is particularly effective at crossing the blood-brain barrier, resulting in a more intense high.

By contrast, inhaled THC undergoes a different metabolic process: Rather than passing through the stomach and then the liver, it travels directly to the brain, which is why the effects of smoked or vaporized marijuana come on faster and diminish more quickly.

Lesson #3: Whoa, That's Potent

Edibles are typically made with highly concentrated cannabis, be it in actual concentrate form (such as hash oil), cannabis-infused butter (cannabutter), or infused oil. This makes it incredibly easy to overdo it. Between the time required for effects to kick in and the high concentrations of THC found in many edibles, finding the correct dose can be tricky. Lindsay's advice: "Consider [a 10-milligram dose] like one beer; this amount will affect some people a lot, and others not at all. Take your time and learn what is right for you."

Consuming too much cannabis can make for a bad experience. Eating the entire canna-cookie may seem like a good idea, but when it comes to edibles, it's best to taste and wait for a while before gorging yourself on potent and delicious treats—particularly because effects take much longer to dissipate than those associated with smoking or vaping.

DID YOU KNOW? Edibles may be strong, but compared to inhaled cannabis, they actually deliver a smaller concentration of cannabinoids to the bloodstream. Ingesting edibles introduces only 10 to 20 percent of THC and other cannabinoids to the blood plasma, whereas inhaled cannabis falls closer to 50 or 60 percent.

Lesson #4: Pay Attention to the Label

Ten milligrams is considered a "dose" in most places where cannabis is legal. However, you'll frequently see products on the market (particularly in medical dispensaries) that contain two or more doses—and sometimes even as many as twenty. Always read the label carefully

DID YOU KNOW? In Colorado's legal marijuana market, 10 milligrams of THC (or CBD) is considered a "standard" dose that normally delivers mild effects. A 100-milligram edible is considered much (much, much) more potent and should be split into several doses over time. Colossal amounts of THC won't kill you, but trust us: You will enjoy the next several hours of your life more if you dose responsibly and patiently.

before you chow down on the whole chocolate bar.

Even after reading the label, there's still some uncertainty as far as the actual dose contained by any given product. A cookie whose label advertises its potency as 10 milligrams may actually contain 8 milligrams, or 13. Generally, this is an honest accident. Because the cannabis industry is in its infancy, manufacturers of edibles are still working out best practices and exact formulas, and thanks to the plant's federal illegality, cannabis products are not yet subject to FDA regulations. Cannabis-testing regulations, which vary widely, are up to individual states, and testing practices are still in their infancy, too. The lack of industry consistency can make finding the correct dose even more difficult. Your best bet is to find a producer that labels products clearly and provides consistent test results, and keep in mind that there may still be a small margin of error that can affect your experience.

Lesson #5: The Effects Are Different

Effects vary between edibles, but generally, consumers report stronger body effects coupled with an almost psychedelic head high in large doses. Smaller amounts yield milder and arguably more comfortable effects. When consumed properly, edibles can offer a wholly unique cannabis experience for recreational consumers, or provide lasting relief for certain medical conditions that other delivery methods can't.

Reasons for choosing edibles over other consumption methods vary, too. Many people become interested in edibles because they don't enjoy the harsh experience of smoking or are worried about long-term health concerns associated with it. Edibles can also oftentimes provide longer-lasting relief for chronic symptoms like pain, often making them a preferred choice for medical patients.

6 TIPS FOR YOUR FIRST TIME DOSING EDIBLES

1. Read the Package Very Carefully
Edibles on the legal market state THC contents in milligrams. The standard dose in most places is 10 milligrams. However, certain products may contain as little as 1 milligram or as many as 200. Never eat anything you're unsure about.

2. Respect Your Tolerance
A cannabis newbie or low-tolerance consumer should start with half a standard dose, or 5 milligrams.

3. Be Patient and Mindful
It's hard to wait for the effects to kick in, but we can't reiterate "start low and go slow" enough. And remember not to snack on that bag of infused gummies when you start to get the munchies—if you lose track of what you're eating, you could be in for a bumpy ride.

4. Don't Dose on an Empty Stomach
Before you eat an edible, have a full meal and drink some water. Edibles kick in faster and come on stronger on an empty stomach.

5. Find a Comfortable Place
Edibles are best consumed in a comfortable setting, such as your home. It's a good idea to have your best friend or partner with you—they can help if you need anything or get nervous.

6. Relax
When consumed responsibly, edibles offer a unique, relaxing, and incredibly enjoyable experience. And if you get higher than you meant to, don't panic— the effects will ebb as time passes and you'll be back to normal before you know it.

Basics of Cooking with Cannabis

The Importance of Decarboxylation

HERE'S A SCENARIO we have all seen in film before: Somebody consumes an entire bag of raw cannabis in order to avoid getting caught with it. Eyes pop wide open and gasps ensue. "You just ate that whole bag!" somebody shouts. However, the aftermath of this scene usually involves a very different representation than what actually happens when you consume raw cannabis. Spoiler alert: The effects will be lackluster at best. Why is this the case?

The answer to this mystery lies in a process called decarboxylation, one that is necessary for us to enjoy the psychoactive effects of the cannabinoids we consume.

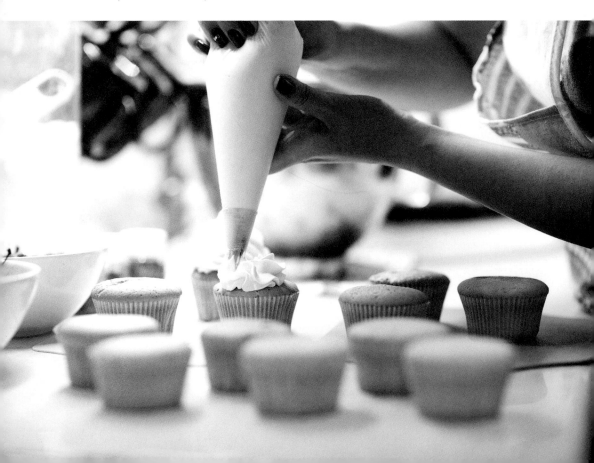

The Basics of Decarboxylation

All cannabinoids contained within the trichomes of raw cannabis flowers have an extra carboxyl ring or group (COOH) attached to their chain. For example, tetrahydrocannabinolic acid (THCA, the nonpsychoactive acid in raw flower that's broken down during decarboxylation to yield the familiar psychoactive THC) is synthesized in prevalence within the trichome heads of freshly harvested cannabis flowers. In most regulated markets, cannabis distributed in dispensaries is labeled detailing the product's cannabinoid contents. THCA, in many cases, prevails as the highest cannabinoid present in products that have not been decarboxylated (e.g., raw cannabis flowers).

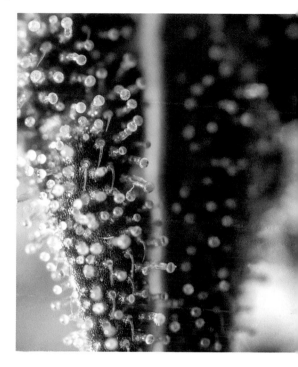

THCA has a number of known benefits when consumed, including anti-inflammatory and neuroprotective qualities. But THCA is not psychoactive, and must be converted into THC through decarboxylation before any effects can be felt.

What Causes Decarboxylation?

The two main catalysts for decarboxylation to occur are heat and time. Drying and curing cannabis over time will cause a partial decarboxylation to occur. This is why some cannabis flowers also test for a presence of small amounts of THC along with THCA. Smoking and vaporizing will instantaneously decarboxylate cannabinoids due to the extremely high temperatures present, making them instantly available for absorption through inhalation.

While decarboxylated cannabinoids in vapor form can be easily absorbed in our lungs, edibles require these cannabinoids to be present in what we consume in order for our bodies to absorb them throughout digestion. Heating cannabinoids at a lower temperature over time allows us to decarboxylate the cannabinoids while preserving the integrity of the material we use so that we may infuse it into what we consume.

At What Temperature Does Decarboxylation Occur?

The THCA in cannabis begins to decarboxylate at approximately 220°F after around thirty to forty-five minutes of exposure. Full decarboxylation may require more time to occur. Many people choose to decarboxylate their cannabis at slightly lower temperatures for a much longer period of time in attempts to preserve terpenes. Many mono- and sesquiterpenes are volatile and will evaporate at higher temperatures, leaving potentially undesirable flavors and aromas behind. The integrity of both cannabinoids and terpenoids are compromised at temperatures that exceed 300°F, which is why temperatures in the 200°F range are recommended.

Heat and time can also cause other forms of cannabinoid degradation to occur. For example, CBN (cannabinol) is formed through the degradation and oxidization of THC, a process that can occur alongside decarboxylation. CBN makes for a much more sedating and less directly psychoactive experience.

How to Decarboxylate Cannabis at Home

In order to decarboxylate cannabis at home, all you need is some starting material, an oven set to 220°F to 235°F (depending on your location and oven model), some parchment paper, and a baking tray. Finely grind your cannabis until the material can be spread thinly over the parchment and placed on your baking sheet. Allow the cannabis to bake for thirty to forty-five minutes, or longer if desired.

Cannabis can also be decarboxylated in a slow cooker by introducing solvents such as cooking oils or lecithin. These methods create infusions that can be used in a variety of recipes, topicals, and even cannabis capsules. Since they contain decarboxylated cannabinoids, they will be effective any way you choose to consume them.

The next time you see somebody on television falling over onto the ground after eating an entire bag of shake, you'll be able to laugh it off over a batch of your very own freshly baked and infused, fully decarboxylated cannabis cookies.

FUN FACT While most semi-experienced consumers can tell the difference between an indica and a sativa strain when vaped, smoked, or dabbed, it's much harder to tell which is which in edible form. Only a few edibles manufacturers label their products as specifically made with indica or sativa strains, and even seasoned consumers are often unable to distinguish between them.

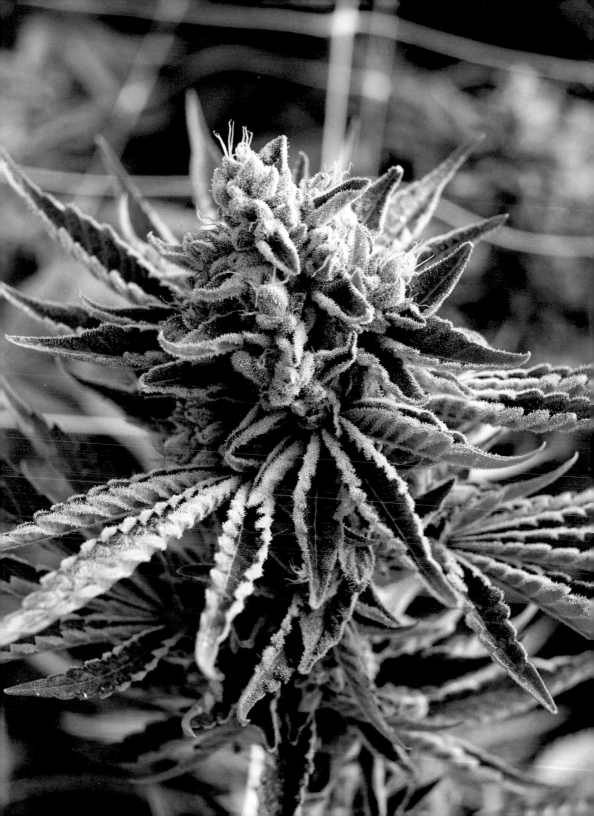

Infused Cooking Advice from Three Pro Cannabis Chefs

Professional cannabis chefs have one of the coolest jobs ever. Then again, it's hard enough to put together a spectacular meal in the kitchen without the added challenge of incorporating the perfect amount and type of cannabis for each dish. How do canna-chefs do it?

To find out, we talked to three of the pros:

Chef Monica Lo, creator of sous-vide cannabis site Sous Weed

Chef Scott Peabody, executive chef at San Francisco's Nomiku

Chef Jose Rodriguez, chef at Google

Q: How does cannabis make you a better cook?

Scott Peabody: Using cannabis as an ingredient (as opposed to merely a psychoactive additive) is especially intriguing to me as a chef because it's still largely uncharted territory. Cooking with cannabis is tricky, because you have to strike a balance between THC extraction and flavor. Remembering that cannabis is, in fact, an herb, I treat it as a culinary challenge like any other, and so it becomes a lesson in restraint and finesse—the skills to strive for, because they separate great cooks from mediocre ones.

Monica Lo: I find that I am a more creative person when lightly medicated and I'm definitely a sativa diva. But more often than not, I make my meals and snacks using raw cannabis for all the wonderful health benefits, not the psychoactive effects. The herbaceous flavors are fairly mild and can be easily incorporated into many dishes. Like Scott mentioned, it's a largely uncharted territory and [it's] fun figuring out how to integrate this ingredient into everyday meals.

Q: What things are important to think about in planning an infused meal?

Peabody: As is the case with anyone who makes cannabis edibles on a small scale, controlling dosage is our single biggest hurdle. Because the guests at our dinners will have a wide range of tolerances, our goal is to accommodate everyone by a) knowing the dose in individual items and keeping it fairly low, and b) serving condiments with a higher dosage, so people can increase their dose ad libitum.

Q: What are your favorite recipes that home cannabis cooks should try?

Lo: Fresh cannabis chimichurri. Raw cannabis is such a nutrient-dense veggie with many beneficial cannabinoids . . . It's also nonpsychoactive before heating so you can enjoy all the health benefits of this miracle plant on top of a juicy skirt steak.

Peabody: Dank dulce de leche. If you want to make anything from banana bread to salted caramel ice cream just a little more cosmic, this is a wonderful ingredient. When done correctly, the cannabis flavor is subtle but pleasant, adding an interesting herbaceous note.

Jose Rodriguez: A cocktail infused with cannabis. Cocktails may not be considered a meal but it's definitely something I like to indulge in while cooking!

Q: What are your favorite munchies, and how do you dress them up?

Lo: Lately I've been indulging in açaí bowls. Açaí, berries, and banana slices are all ingredients I keep in my freezer and all I need to do is dump it into my Vitamix with some coconut water and honey then puree until smooth. I top it off with some crunchy granola and toasted coconut chips. This sometimes doubles as my dinner while I'm binge-watching television.

Peabody: My answer has to be spaghetti alla carbonara, which needs no dressing up. Though many Americans mistakenly think of it as fancy restaurant fodder, natives of Rome, where the dish originates, often eat carbonara as the ideal midnight snack, to be indulged in after a night of revelry. It's quick and easy to make, and I almost always have all the necessary ingredients on hand: Parmigiano (or pecorino), guanciale (or bacon), eggs, and dry pasta. Embrace the low-key fanciness. Runner-up option (if I'm too high to make carbonara) is popcorn, which I typically dress up by adding finely grated cheese (such as aged cheddar or Gruyère) and chili flakes.

Rodriguez: I must agree on popcorn but I prefer it with caramel.

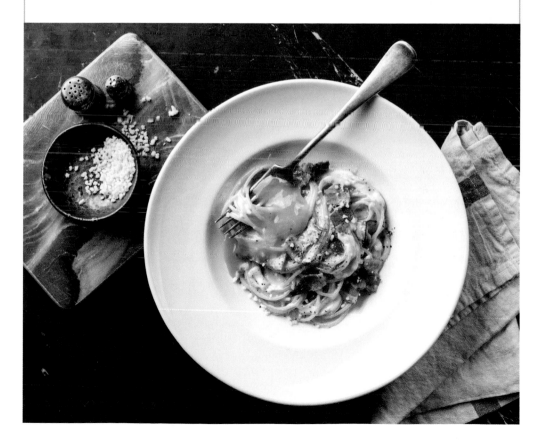

Dosing Homemade Edibles

Why It's Nearly Impossible to Calculate Potency

HERE AT LEAFLY, we once held a bake-off to determine the best pot brownie recipe of all time. In our competition, each recipe called for varying amounts of cannabutter, canna-oil, or in one case, ground raw cannabis flower (bold move, Mario Batali). So once the brownies were baked, we set out to calculate the potency of each batch. Seemed like we'd just need to dust off our basic math skills, right? Well, we were wrong. Calculating potency, it turns out, is easier in theory than in practice. So we got in touch with Dr. Kymron deCesare, chief research officer at cannabis testing facility Steep Hill Labs, to figure out what was going on.

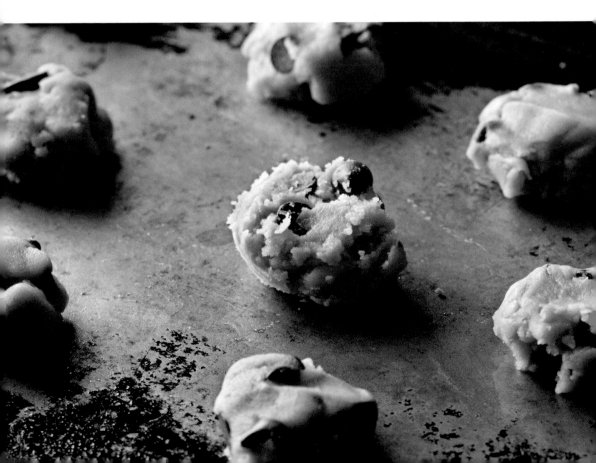

What's Going On During the Cooking Process?

DeCesare explains that it's extremely difficult to get an accurate analysis of the amount of cannabinoids in an edible, even a professionally made one. In fact, it's so tricky that licensed edibles producers have to test their products at multiple stages. First, they test the cannabis flowers to be used in the production run. This initial analysis provides an estimate of how much of each cannabinoid and terpene is available for extraction. Subsequent testing of the extract determines how effective the extraction process actually was. Finally, testing of the spent plant matter post extraction confirms the amount of cannabinoids and terpenoids left behind. Home bakers, however, lack the resources to pursue these types of analyses.

"Because of the excessive amount of time required to extract, we normally see a lot of damage done to the primary drugs of interest," including THC, CBD, and various terpenes, says deCesare. This is particularly true if you plan to bake your edibles at temperatures over 300°F, at which point some compounds (particularly terpenes) begin to burn off. What's lost in the extraction and baking process? For one thing, a given amount of THCA does not convert to an equivalent amount of THC: Rather, the conversion rate is 0.88. While many producers will do this conversion for you and note the potential amount of THC in a given strain on the packaging, some denote only the percentage of THCA present, which adds an extra step to the calculations.

Then there's the inefficiency of butter and oil extraction. "For clients that normally extract into dairy butterfat, they discover they only extracted between 40 and 60 percent of the cannabinoids and terpenoids," explains deCesare. Lena Davidson of Botanica, one of Washington State's largest edibles producers, puts the estimate even lower, at close to 30 percent. Davidson adds that certain oils are even less effective at extraction: In general, butter and coconut oil are the most ideal extractors, while others like canola and vegetable oil retain even fewer cannabinoids.

Overall, "the only way to know for sure [how potent your homemade edible is] would be to have the butter analyzed so you know exactly how much THC is in it," says deCesare. Davidson argues that even this testing has yielded inaccurate results for Botanica in the past. "We learned really early on that we couldn't rely on a butter potency test," she says. Botanica has since shifted to testing individual products from every batch.

Tips for Reducing Variation in Edibles Dosing

The difficulty of accurately determining edible potency is staggering even on a professional scale, so it's no surprise that accurately dosing your own edibles at home is all but impossible. That said, the following are some best practices that can help hobby bakers minimize the inevitable variance in the potency of their homemade edibles.

▪ *Check the label before you extract.* Some producers note THC on flower packaging, while others note THCA. If you see a THCA percentage, use the 0.88 conversion rate to determine potential THC.

▪ *Portion cannabutter vertically.* "Gravity impacts everything," says Davidson, "and each cannabinoid has a different molecular weight, so they will settle in different places." Butter from the bottom of the batch will be different than butter from the top, so don't scoop straight off the top.

▪ *Measure carefully.* Don't plop a big spoonful of cannabutter into the batter—get out the measuring cups, and fill and level them precisely.

▪ *Stir well.* DeCesare says that "unless you quantitatively measured out consistent [cannabutter] portions into each and every brownie . . . you have another contributing error in the final product." The next best thing is to stir until you're positive the batter is perfectly homogenous—and then stir some more.

▪ *Portion uniformly.* Don't attack the brownie pan with a fork; cut into equal pieces (using a ruler can help). Cookies are even harder; use a kitchen scale to weigh out equal portions of dough.

▪ *Plan on variation.* Use our potency estimation example to calculate the maximum potential cannabinoids in your edibles. When in doubt, assume that the maximum amount of THC made it into your final product; you can always eat more later if you find you were wrong.

Example of an Edible Potency Estimation

1. I have 100 g of top-shelf Sour Diesel. I know that top shelf is always approximately 20 percent, or 200mg THCA per 1 g of flower. 200 mg x 100 = 20,000 mg THCA.

2. The conversation from THCA to THC is 0.88. 20,000 mg x 0.88 = 17,600 mg maximum THC available to be extracted.

3. Under ideal conditions, you get a 60 percent efficiency of extraction in dairy butter, so 17,600 mg x 0.6 = 10,560 mg maximum THC likely to be extracted.

4. If my targeted dosage is 200 mg per brownie, then 10,560 mg / 200 = 53 brownies containing 200 mg each. This is the absolute maximum those brownies will have; they will likely contain a whole lot less depending on cumulative errors.

Make Your Own Cannabutter at Home

CANNABIS-INFUSED BUTTER (CAN- NABUTTER) is one of the simplest and most common ways to make medicated foods, yet making infused butter properly can be a little bit tricky. In order for THC to properly decarboxylate— change from its acid form to its psychoactive form—the cannabis must be heated at low temperatures over long periods of time.

We recommend simmering your cannabis either on the stove or in a slow cooker at a temperature range of 225°F to 250°F for a long period of time. This will ensure that your cannabis does not become too hot too quickly and burn off active cannabinoids.

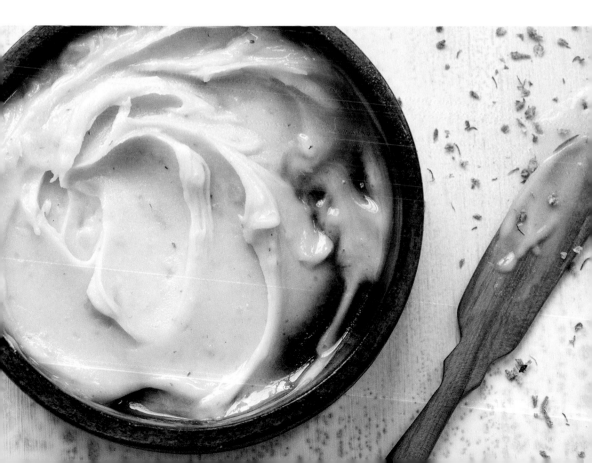

Two Variations for Making Cannabis-Infused Butter (Cannabutter)

Ingredients

1 pound unsalted butter

1 cup water (add more water at any time if needed)

1 ounce of ground cannabis flower or 1½ ounces of high-quality cannabis trim (this amount will make some pretty potent butter, so decrease the amount of cannabis if you want a recipe that delivers lighter doses)

Note: Some people also use the remnants of vaporized cannabis to make cannabutter, as many vaporizers fail to decarboxylate all of the THC in flower.

Stove-Top Method:

1. Add butter and water to a stockpot or saucepan; let the butter melt and begin to simmer on low. Adding water helps to regulate the temperature and prevents the butter from scorching.

2. As butter begins to melt, add in your ground cannabis product.

3. Maintain low heat and let the mixture simmer for 2 to 3 hours, stirring occasionally. Make sure the mixture never comes to a full boil.

Slow-Cooker Method (Our Personal Favorite):

1. Turn slow cooker onto low; add butter, water, and ground cannabis flower.

2. Cover slow cooker and let simmer on low for 8 to 24 hours, stirring occasionally. When it comes to infusing butter, the longer you let the cannabis product simmer, the more cannabinoids will be infused into the final product.

For Both Methods:

1. After simmering for your desired amount of time, pour the hot mixture into a glass, refrigerator-safe container, using cheesecloth or fine-mesh strainer to strain out all plant product from the butter mixture. Squeeze or press the plant material to get as much liquid off of the plant product as possible. Discard leftover plant material.

2. Cover and refrigerate remaining liquid overnight or until the butter is fully hardened. Once hardened, the butter will separate from the water, allowing you to lift the now infused cannabutter from the water to use in your recipes. Discard remaining water after removing the hardened cannabutter.

3. Let the cannabutter sit at room temperature to soften for use. Do not use a microwave to soften the butter.

How to Make Cannabis Cooking Oil (Canna-Oil)

ALONGSIDE CANNABUTTER, CANNABIS-INFUSED oil is one of the most versatile mediums for infused cooking, since it can be used for baking desserts, sautéing veggies, frying up your morning eggs, or in your salad dressing. The method for making it is comparable to cannabutter.

Oils with the highest fat content will be more effective in activating the THC. Coconut and olive oil are probably the most common choices; coconut oil has a milder taste and can therefore be used in more dishes, whereas olive oil is the staple cooking oil for most kitchens. However, both have trouble with high heat, in which case canola oil may make the most sense.

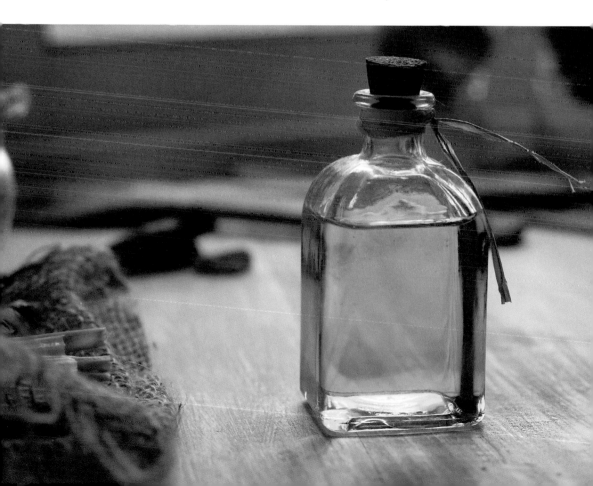

Cannabis Cooking Oil

Ingredients:

1 ounce cannabis flower (or less for milder potency)

2 cups cooking oil of your choice (see p. 133)

Directions:

1. Grind the cannabis. You can include the entire plant, just the flower, a little bit of both—this is all a matter of preference.

2. Combine oil and cannabis in your pan of choice, and heat the two together on low for hours. This allows for decarboxylation (activation of THC) without scorching, which destroys the active ingredients. Like with cannabutter, cooking can be done a variety of ways: in a slow cooker on low for up to three days (minimum of 6 hours), stirring occasionally; in a double boiler on low for at least 6 hours (8 is better), stirring occasionally; or in a simple saucepan on low for at least 3 hours, stirring frequently (a saucepan is most susceptible to scorching). In all cases, a small amount of water can be added to the mixture to help avoid burning.

3. Strain and store the oil. All remaining plant material can be discarded or used in other dishes if you have the wherewithal. The oil's shelf life is at least 2 months, and can be extended with refrigeration.

> **Note:** Be cautious when using the oil to prepare dishes that require heating. Do not microwave, and choose low heat whenever possible.

PRO TIP Many experienced cannabis chefs like to use the entire cannabis plant, in part for conservation but also for the health benefits the more fibrous parts of the plants have been linked to. Just keep in mind that the more inactive parts of the plant that are included, the stronger the cannabis flavor, and that anything small enough to fit through your strainer will end up in your finished product.

Cannabis Tinctures

How to Make Them and How to Use Them

CANNABIS TINCTURES, ALSO known as green or golden dragon, are alcohol-based cannabis extracts—essentially, infused alcohol. In fact, tinctures were the main form of cannabis medicine until the United States enacted cannabis prohibition. With a name like "green dragon," you might think cannabis tinctures are not for the faint of heart, but they're actually a great entry point for both recreational and medical users looking to ease into smokeless consumption methods.

How to Dose and Use Cannabis Tinctures

Tincture dosages are easy to self-titrate, or measure. Start with one milliliter of your finished tincture and put it under your tongue. If you're happy with the effects, you're done. Otherwise, try two milliliters the next day and so on until you find the volume you're happy with (ramp up slowly while testing your desired dosage so you can avoid getting uncomfortably high).

Tinctures will last for many years when stored in a cool, dark location. When combined with easy self-titration, the long shelf life means you can make larger quantities of tinctures at once and have a convenient, accurate way to ingest cannabis.

Compared to the traditional cannabis-infused brownie, tinctures are a low calorie alternative. If you make your tincture with 190-proof alcohol, you're looking at about 7 calories per milliliter. Unless you have an extremely weak

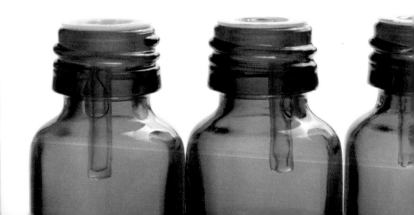

tincture, you'll easily stay under your typical brownie's 112 calorie count (and let's face it, your brownies are probably far more caloric than that).

Tinctures can be incorporated after cooking into all sorts of meals and drinks:

- Juices
- Ice creams and sherbets
- Soups
- Gelatin
- Mashed potatoes and gravy
- Salad dressing

How to Make Cannabis Tinctures

If you don't have a well-equipped kitchen or just prefer simple, mess-free preparation techniques, cannabis tinctures are a great DIY project. At a minimum, you can make a tincture with a jar, alcohol, a strainer, and cannabis flower. That's all you need!

Depending on your available time, equipment, and risk tolerance, you'll prefer some of the following recipes over others.

Traditional Green Dragon

If you've heard about green dragon before, this is probably the recipe you're most familiar with.

1. Decarboxylate your flower or extract (if you're using flower, grind it to a fine consistency).

2. Mix your flower or extract in a mason jar with high-proof alcohol (preferably Everclear).

3. Close the jar and let it sit for two to three weeks, shaking it once a day.

4. After a few weeks, pour it through a coffee filter, discarding the solids. Start with a small dose of 1 milliliter to assess potency.

Master Wu's Green Dragon

This recipe was first published in 2006 on cannabis.com and is one of the most comprehensive tincture recipes available online, with detailed instructions and excellent tips and tricks. Master Wu's recipe differs from the traditional method in that it uses heat to speed up the extraction and concentration process. Unlike the traditional method, you'll be finished with this recipe in an evening.

1. Decarboxylate your flower or extract (if you're using flower, grind it to a fine consistency).

2. Mix your flower or extract in a mason jar with high-proof alcohol (preferably Everclear).

3. Simmer the jar in a water bath for 20 minutes at 170°F.

4. Strain the mixture and store.

Modern Green Dragon

If you're following some of the latest developments in online tincture recipes, you may have heard of the following recipe. It sounds too good to be true, but many people (including myself) are having great results with it.

1. Decarboxylate your flower or extract (if you're using flower, grind it to a fine consistency).

2. Mix your flower or extract in a mason jar with high-proof alcohol (preferably Everclear).

3. Shake for 3 minutes.

4. Strain the mixture and store.

CANNABIS TINCTURE FAQS

How do I take my tincture?

Tinctures are usually taken by putting a few drops under your tongue (sublingually). When taken this way, the arterial blood supply under your tongue rapidly absorbs the THC. That being said, you can always swallow the tincture in a drink or food, but it will be absorbed more slowly by your liver.

How fast is the onset?

When dosing a tincture sublingually, expect to feel the effects in 15 to 45 minutes and reach your peak high at about 90 minutes. If you simply drink the dose, expect a slower onset that more closely resembles traditional edibles.

How long will I feel the effects?

Expect to be high longer than when you smoke or vaporize, but shorter than when you eat a butter- or oil-based edible.

Pairing Food and Drinks with Cannabis

A Primer

CANNABIS AND FOOD: two substances with the power to make people very happy. Few things make a better pair, and with thousands of cannabis strains and the entire world of food and drink at our disposal, more pairings are possible today than ever before. The question is: How to go about matching a dish or beverage with its perfect cannabis counterpart?

Regardless of whether you're a wine-and-cheese pro or completely uninitiated to the process, don't be intimidated by pairings—they're easier than you think.

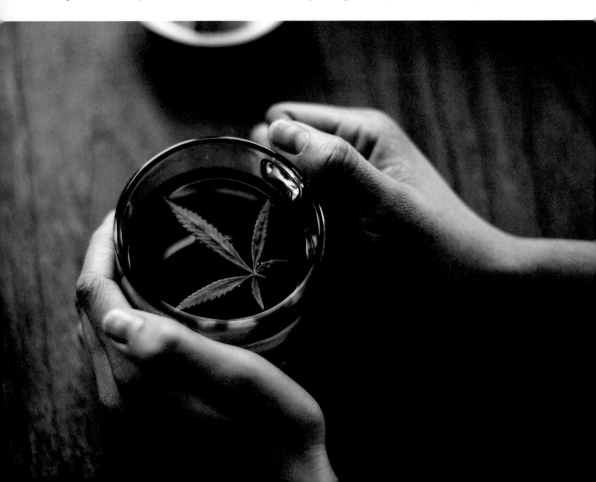

Basic Tenets of Cannabis Pairing

No matter what you're matching it with, the right cannabis pairing starts with an understanding of cannabis terpenes—the naturally occurring compounds that give individual strains their unique aromas and flavors. Terpenes are found in varying concentrations in different cannabis strains, with all strains containing at least a few different terpenes. Myrcene, for instance, is what gives Jillybean its tropical fruit flavor; a high concentration of pinene imparts a foresty flavor profile to Jack Herer.

Matching these aroma and flavor profiles with other aromas and flavors that complement or accentuate them is what makes for a great pairing. Say you're trying a new salmon recipe for dinner, and the recipe calls for a squeeze of lemon juice. A lemony strain, such as Super Lemon Haze, will help highlight those lemon flavors in the dish. Conversely, say you've made lemon bars for dessert; with plenty of lemon flavor packed into each bar, you might choose a complementarily flavored strain, like Blueberry, to balance out that intense citrusy sweetness.

Whether you choose comparable or contrasting flavors is up to you—there are no right or wrong answers, and pairing is all about personal preference. Do you like the pairing? Then it's a good one. Just as everyone experiences the effects of different cannabis strains a little bit differently, everyone (even the pros) experiences flavors a little bit differently, too. Factors including body chemistry, past experiences, and the region you're in can all affect what you taste, so don't waste time worrying about whether you're doing it right.

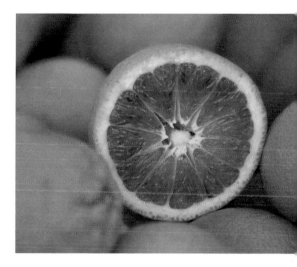

How to Get Started

If you're a beginner, cannabis strains with high terpene levels are a great place to start; they'll have the most pronounced aromas and flavors, which make them easier to match. Your budtender will be able to guide you toward strains with high levels of terpenes (between 2 and 4 percent total terpene content is generally considered high). Take a whiff of the flower and consider what you smell. Is it sweet? Citrusy? Spicy? Now, think about what foods or drinks those flavors would go well with. Sticking your nose in a jar of peppery Power Plant may inspire you to whip up some lemon-pepper chicken. With citrus-laden Tangie, your first thought may be a big glass of iced tea.

Descriptively named strains can also clue you in to potential pairings. Agent Orange, for instance, is so named for its juicy orange aroma and flavor, so think of foods or drinks that might naturally be complemented by an orange slice, such as teriyaki chicken or a summery Hefeweizen. Browse strains by flavor at leafly.com/start-exploring.

When pairing, the best means of consuming the strain you've selected is with a vaporizer compatible with cannabis flower. Vaporization lets terpene flavors shine through without burning them off like combustion does; you can even customize which terpenes you're inhaling by tweaking the temperature settings on more advanced machines.

Regardless of your experience level, there's simply no substitute for practice (good thing; that's the fun part). Pairing is far from an exact science, so the most important thing is to play around enough so you learn what you like. Whenever you

FUN FACT Terpenes are present in food, too: You'll find them providing aromas, flavors, and health benefits in everything from oranges and tomatoes to seafood and herbs.

try a new pairing, be sure to write down whether you liked it so you can learn from your experiences.

The following are a few basic pairings; use them to get you started, then strike out on your own!

- *Spinach Strawberry Salad* with *Blue Dream*. A fresh, farmer's market-inspired salad, particularly one with sliced berries, is only made better by this juicy, berry-forward hybrid.

- *Hawaiian Pizza* and *Pineapple Express*. Everyone knows the pineapple chunks on a slice of Hawaiian pizza are the best part. Pair each bite with a hit of sweet, tropical Pineapple Express to highlight that flavor.

- *Chocolate Chip Cookies* with *Sour Diesel*. Offset the sweetness of this classic dessert with the pungent, earthy flavor of Sour Diesel.

One more great thing about cannabis pairings is that cannabinoids—particularly THC—will heighten your enjoyment of flavors, textures, and colors in most any food or drink. To make the most of your pairings, try choosing dishes that exhibit rich flavors, bright colors, and unique textures. Furthermore, most cannabis strains augment our desire to chow down (hence the munchies), so it's hard to go wrong with whatever you decide to cook up or snack on.

Pairing Cannabis with Beverages

When pairing cannabis with beverages, particularly alcoholic ones, there is another element to consider in addition to flavor: how the effects of the cannabis pair with the effects of the beverage. This additional layer to the pairing process makes it a little more challenging but also a lot of fun.

Indicas, sativas, and hybrids can beget a wide range of effects: Some strains are uplifting and euphoric, while others are relaxed and sleepy. The best pairings consider both the flavors of each individual constituent and how the effects of one will offset or accentuate the effects of the other. If you're holding a Russian imperial stout with 12 percent alcohol by volume, you should probably steer clear of potent, body-heavy indicas like Granddaddy Purple, unless you want to end up napping all afternoon in an armchair (though that can be enjoyable, too). On the other hand, pairing an after-dinner espresso with an energetic sativa might be a recipe for disaster if you don't want to be up all night—so consider switching your strain choice, or brewing a shot of decaf.

> **Remember:** With pairing cannabis with alcohol, it is all the more imperative that you consume legally and responsibly. Always practice moderation, and never drive under the influence of THC, alcohol, or both.

Leafly's Top 10 Cannabis-Infused Recipes

ONCE YOU KNOW how to make cannabutter, cannabis-infused cooking oils, and cannabis tinctures, the world is your oyster when it comes to infused recipes. You can substitute part or all of the butter or oil in any standard recipe to make a medicated version, and you can just as easily add a few drops of tincture to any drink you like. That said, it's a great idea to start with recipes created using infused ingredients until you get used to making homemade edibles. The following recipes are some of our all-time favorites.

When you're working with homemade recipes, be sure to start with just a little butter, oil, or tincture until you're confident with its potency; you can always increase the serving size or make a stronger batch later.

Find more infused recipes and cooking tips at Leafly.com.

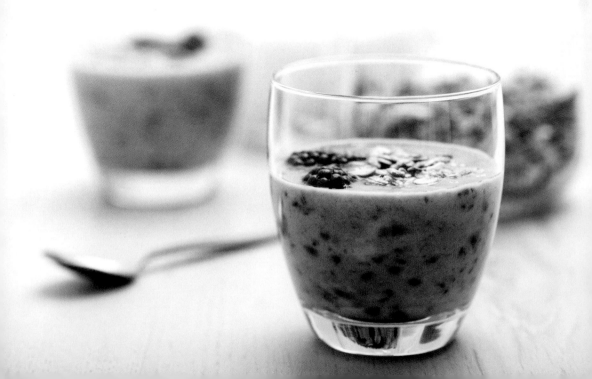

Raw Cannabis Breakfast Smoothie

Rise and shine with the superpower of cannabis! Raw cannabis is naturally loaded with powerful antioxidants that fight disease, reduce inflammation, and repair damaged cells.

Combining the forces of raw cannabis, hemp seeds, and hemp milk, this nonpsychoactive smoothie is the perfect balance of breakfast fuels to start your day off right.

½ cup hemp milk

1 tablespoon hemp seeds

1 teaspoon flax seeds

½ cup chopped green kale

¼ cup sliced cucumber

2 slices cantaloupe

1 banana

Fresh raw cannabis (about ½ cup)

1. Place all the ingredients in a blender. Add water and ice to taste.

2. Blend until smooth, pour into a glass and enjoy! Makes two 8-ounce servings.

Wake 'n' Bake Granola

With a prolonged delivery and lengthy duration, morning edibles (when managed correctly) can offer a steady, gradual lift to your day that many habitual consumers cherish. One satisfying and nourishing option is this cannabis-infused granola. It's fabulous on its own as a small snack or atop your favorite yogurt for a power-packed parfait.

¼ cup almonds, soaked in water for over an hour

¼ cup sunflower seeds

¼ cup walnuts, soaked

4 fresh dates

¼ teaspoon ground cinnamon

Pinch of salt

2 doses cannabis-infused cooking oil

1. Preheat the oven to 250°F.

2. Blend the nuts and seeds in a food processor until coarsely chopped.

3. Add the dates and blend into a paste.

4. Place the date and nut mixture in a medium bowl with the cinnamon, salt, and oil. Mix everything together.

5. Line a glass dish with parchment paper and spread the mix into a thin layer on top of the parchment.

6. Bake 18 minutes, or until the top turns a golden brown.

7. Let cool or refrigerate to allow the granola to adhere and solidify.

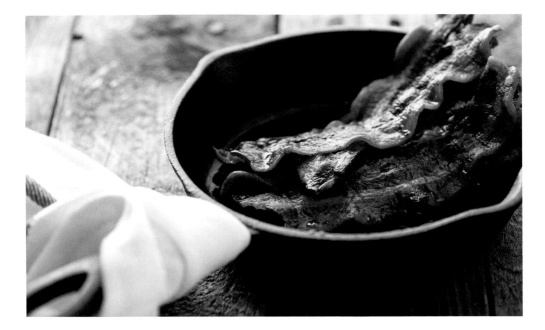

Canna-Bacon

Just when you think you've experienced all there is to love about bacon, you learn about cannabis-infused bacon. Aside from the marvel that is the union of these two royalties, the real ingenuity lies in utilizing the bacon fat for activation of the THC in the cannabis.

2 grams cannabis, ground into a fine powder (use less for reduced potency)

1 (16-ounce) package sliced bacon

1. Preheat oven to 225°F. Spread the ground cannabis onto a cookie sheet and bake for 45 minutes to decarboxylate.

2. Place the bacon strips on an ungreased cookie sheet.

3. Once the cannabis is done baking, remove and raise the oven temperature to 275°F. Sprinkle half of the baked cannabis over each strip of bacon, adding more or less depending on the desired potency.

4. Bake the bacon for 10 minutes. Remove from oven, flip the strips, and sprinkle more cannabis over the other side. Bake for another 10 minutes. Enjoy!

Note: All leftover fat on the cookie sheet is medicinally active, so you may want to save it and get creative! One quick option is to soak up the grease with bread and *voilà:* cannabis bacon bread. You can also use it as an oil substitute for egg scrambles, stir-fries, and more.

Guaca-Holy-Mole

THC is fat-soluble, not water-soluble, meaning it's necessary to fuse cannabis with fattier foods to capture the THC and yield the herb's medicinal benefits. Packed with plenty of healthy fat, avocados could be categorized as the perfect ingredient for preparing cannabis edibles.

4 grams cannabis, ground into a fine powder

4 avocados, peeled, pitted, and mashed

Juice of 2 limes

1 small red onion, diced

⅓ cup cilantro, finely chopped

2 Roma tomatoes, chopped

1 clove garlic, minced

Add-ins (optional):

Freshly ground black pepper

Finely ground sea salt

Cayenne pepper

Diced chiles (such as serrano or jalapeño)

1. Preheat oven to 225°F. Spread the ground cannabis on a cookie sheet and bake for 45 minutes to decarboxylate.

2. In a medium bowl, mix together the remaining ingredients. Stir in the baked cannabis.

3. Adjust with optional add-ins until the desired spice level and seasoning is reached.

4. Cover with plastic wrap and refrigerate for at least 1 hour before serving.

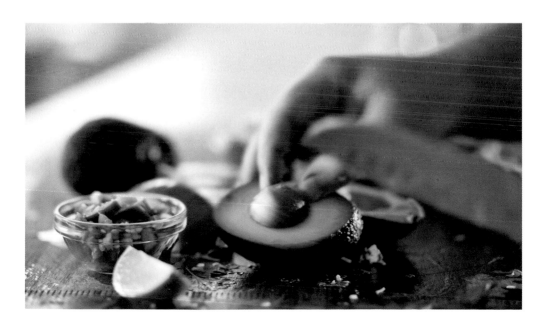

Creamy Canna–Mashed Potatoes

These creamy, tasty taters are perfect for your holiday table, or as comfort food all year round. The cannabutter lends a beautiful herbaceous note that's offset by the rich, garlicky dish.

5 pounds Yukon gold potatoes, peeled

2 (3-ounce) packages cream cheese

¼ cup cannabutter (use less for reduced potency)

¼ cup unsalted butter

½ cup sour cream

¼ cup milk

1½ teaspoons garlic powder

Ground white pepper to taste

1 teaspoon fresh rosemary, chopped (optional)

1. Place the potatoes in a large pot of lightly salted water. Bring to a boil, and cook until tender, 15 to 20 minutes. Drain and mash.

2. While the potatoes are still warm, in a large bowl, combine the mashed potatoes with the cream cheese, cannabutter, regular butter, sour cream, milk, garlic powder, and pepper, and blend until smooth.

3. Sprinkle the rosemary on top (if using), serve, and enjoy! Makes 10 to 12 servings.

"Besto Pesto" Cannabis Pizza

Cannabis-infused pizza sauce is a great way to medicate for several reasons:

- The infused pesto sauce is only one of many distinct ingredients, which means a muted cannabis flavor.
- Pizza is great for sharing, and each slice should provide roughly the same dosage.
- The sky's the limit when it comes to toppings.
- Pizza, you say? Party!

Pesto

1 cup canna-oil

2 cups basil

2 cloves garlic

¼ cup Parmesan cheese

Salt to taste

Pizza

Pizza dough for one regular-sized pizza, rolled out

1 medium tomato, sliced

Goat cheese, crumbled

Mozzarella, shredded

Red peppers, diced

1. Preheat oven to 300°F.

2. Puree all the pesto ingredients in a food processor. (If the potency of the cannabis oil is on the high end, mix half conventional oil and half cannabis oil to make a whole cup.)

3. Spread pesto over pizza dough and add the tomatoes, cheeses, and peppers (or use your favorite toppings). Cook the pizza until browned, on medium-low heat (at a temperature less than 300°F to avoid vaporizing the majority of the cannabinoids).

4. Party on!

Braised Cannabis-Infused Vegetable Medley

When prepared properly, vegetables are delicious and do your body good. No one regrets eating vegetables. Together, veggies and cannabis make this recipe a one-two punch for wellness.

2½ tablespoons cannabis-infused olive oil (use less for reduced potency)

8 small purple potatoes, quartered

1 medium cauliflower, cored, cut into 1-inch florets

3 cloves garlic, minced

¼ teaspoon hot red pepper flakes

1 (14.5 ounce) can diced tomatoes

2 teaspoons minced fresh basil leaves or 1 teaspoon dried basil

1 teaspoon salt

¼ teaspoon Old Bay seasoning (optional)

1. Heat 2 tablespoons of the oil in a large skillet over a medium-high flame.

2. Add the potatoes and cook, stirring occasionally, until they begin to brown and soften slightly, about 15 minutes.

3. Add the cauliflower and continuing to cook, stirring occasionally, until the florets begin to brown, 6 to 7 minutes.

4. Clear a space in the center of the pan and add the garlic, pepper flakes, and remaining oil.

5. Mash and stir the garlic mixture in the center of the pan until it becomes fragrant, about 1 minute. Stir the garlic mixture into the cauliflower and potatoes and cook an additional minute.

6. Add the tomatoes, cover, and cook until cauliflower is tender, but still offers some resistance, 7 to 10 minutes.

7. Add the basil and season with the salt and Old Bay (if using) to taste. Serve immediately and enjoy!

The Best Fudgy Pot Brownies

One of our editors here at Leafly contends that his mom has the best brownie recipe in the universe, so we put it to the test as a cannabis-infused brownie. We love it because it incorporates raspberries, which give it a juicy fruit flavor and pops of rose-red color.

1⅛ cups cannabutter

½ cup 70% cocoa dark chocolate, coarsely chopped

2 cups sugar

4 eggs

1 teaspoon vanilla extract

1 cup all-purpose flour

¼ cup Dutch cocoa powder

½ teaspoon salt

1½ cups raspberries, fresh or frozen (optional)

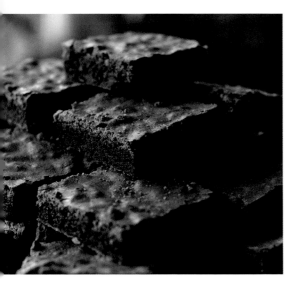

1. Preheat oven to 350°F.

2. Lightly grease a 9 x 9-inch square cake tin. Line with baking paper, extending the paper beyond the rim of the tin. (This makes it easier to get the brownies out later.)

3. Heat the cannabutter in a saucepan over low heat. When half melted, add the chocolate and stir with a wooden spoon until the butter and chocolate are completely melted and combined.

4. Remove from heat and stir in the sugar. Beat in the eggs, one at a time, until mixture is shiny. Stir in the vanilla.

5. Sift in the dry ingredients and mix thoroughly.

6. Pour into prepared tin and top with raspberries (if using).

7. Bake for 35 minutes if not using raspberries and 40 minutes if using raspberries. Do not overcook.

8. Cool completely in the tin.

9. Refrigerate and, once cold, remove from tin and cut into rectangles. Serve chilled!

Cannabis Sugar Cookies

Pop quiz: Which of the following most closely matches your opinion of December?

a) It's the most wonderful time of the year.

b) It's the most stressful time of the year.

c) It's the best time of the year for cookies.

d) All of the above.

If you selected a), b), c), or d), you're in luck! We have the perfect cookie recipe for relishing and relaxing at once. Bake up a batch of these classic sugar cookies infused with a healthy dose of cannabutter. They're easy, festive, delicious, and perfect for delivering a body high at a busy time of year.

1 cup cannabutter (use less for reduced potency)

1 cup sugar

1 egg

1 teaspoon vanilla extract

2½ cups all-purpose flour, plus more for rolling

1 teaspoon baking powder

1 teaspoon salt

Powdered sugar, milk, food coloring for frosting (optional)

1. Beat the cannabutter, sugar, egg, and vanilla in a large bowl on medium speed until thoroughly combined.

2. In a separate bowl, mix together the dry ingredients.

3. Add the dry ingredients to the cannabutter mixture a little at a time, stirring until all ingredients are incorporated.

4. Cover the dough and refrigerate for 1 hour or longer.

5. Preheat the oven to 375° F.

6. Roll the dough on a generously floured surface until it is approximately ⅓-inch thick. Cut cookies and transfer to ungreased baking sheets.

7. Bake for 10 to 12 minutes or until lightly golden in color.

8. Remove from the oven, transfer to cooling rack, and let cool completely before frosting. Yields approximately 2 dozen cookies.

9. To frost, combine powdered sugar with milk and stir until desired consistency is reached, then add food coloring as desired. If you like, add 1 to 2 teaspoons of cannabutter to thicken the frosting and add an extra kick of potency.

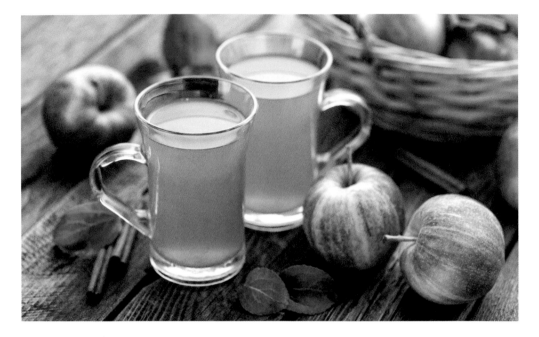

Homemade Tincture-Infused Apple Cider

This sweet seasonal sipper is perfect when the weather cools down, be it on an autumn afternoon or over a holiday break with family and friends. Plus, it's easy to dose; just adjust the amount of tincture you use to suit your needs.

4 to 5 Granny Smith apples

½ cup granulated sugar

¼ cup light brown sugar

2 tablespoons ground cinnamon

1 tablespoon ground allspice

Pinch of grated nutmeg

1 dose glycerin cannabis tincture per serving (recipe serves 3 to 4; adjust based on desired potency)

1. Cut the apples into quarters (don't remove peel or seeds).

2. Place the apples into a large pot and fill with enough water to cover.

3. Add both of the sugars, the cinnamon, allspice, and nutmeg.

4. Boil for 1 hour, uncovered. Check frequently.

5. Cover the pot and turn down the heat and simmer for 2 more hours.

6. Take off the heat and let cool.

7. Mash the apples to a pulp.

8. Once cool, pour into a fine-mesh strainer or cheesecloth over a large bowl. When most of the juice has been strained, squeeze until no more juice comes out.

9. Add the cannabis tincture, stir, and serve.

3 Reasons to Consider Cooking Your Edibles Sous Vide

Sous vide is a method of cooking wherein food is sealed in plastic bags or canning jars and cooked using a water bath held to a specific temperature. With the advent of consumer-grade sous-vide machines, getting started with this method has never been easier, and a precisely heated water bath is wonderful for both decarboxylating your main ingredient and infusing your cooking oil or butter. But why should you consider switching from the classic approach?

1. Sous vide offers precise (and easy) temperature control.

One of the biggest concerns while infusing canna-oil is the temperature: If it's too cool, the THC will bind to the oil at a diminished rate (or not bind at all), and if it's too hot, you're vaporizing some of the psychoactive ingredients and losing potency. Unlike a saucepan, slow cooker, or double boiler, with a sous vide you simply input a temperature on the digital display, and your oil with remain within 1°F of the chosen temperature for the entire cooking duration. This eliminates worry over ruining your top-shelf bud with a temperature-related accident; plus, once you've found a recipe that works, you'll be able to reproduce it perfectly every time.

2. Sous vide is hands-free and low stress.

Infusing oil can be an all-day process that requires some amount of attention throughout. With sous vide, you won't have to babysit the infusion at all—simply keep the water covered with plastic wrap or Ping-Pong balls to prevent evaporation. If you feel comfortable leaving a slow cooker unattended in your house, you can also feel comfortable leaving your sous vide unattended, affording you time to do other, more important things.

3. Sous vide is courteous and covert.

Decarbing flower in your oven and infusing oil on your stovetop can make your kitchen smell a bit dank, which is less than ideal when you have neighbors with sensitive noses or if you want to keep your cannabis use private. Well, it turns out that when you cook your cannabis in an airtight, sealed container that's also under water, there's not a whole lot to smell, which means you can whip up a delicious batch of infused goodies without stinking up your kitchen.

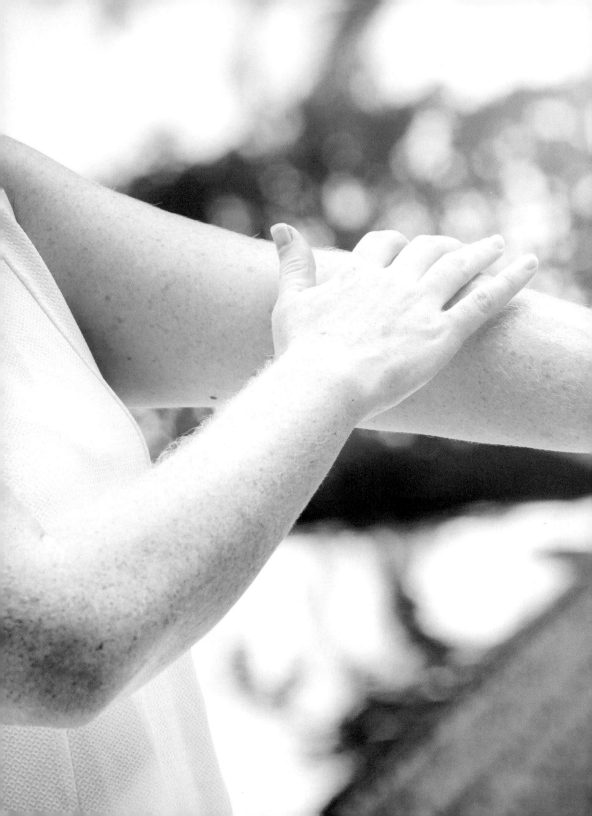

CANNABIS TOPICALS

Topicals (n): Cannabis-infused lotions, oils, body butters, balms, and patches that allow cannabinoids to be absorbed through the skin for relief from pain, swelling, and muscle soreness. Topicals' effects are localized and nonpsychoactive, and can help address conditions as diverse as psoriasis, cramps, and eczema.

Cannabis Topicals 101

NEW METHODS OF cannabis consumption are bringing us farther away from the notion that marijuana belongs solely in a bong or joint—or that it has to get you high, for that matter. Cannabis-infused topicals are an example of how new modes of consumption are revolutionizing perceptions of cannabis as their accessibility, safety, and efficacy invite even the most unlikely patrons into the world of medical marijuana.

What Are Topicals?

Topicals are cannabis-infused lotions, balms, and oils that are absorbed through the skin for localized relief of pain, soreness, and inflammation. Because they're nonpsychoactive, topicals are often chosen by patients who want the therapeutic benefits of marijuana without the cerebral euphoria associated with other delivery methods. Other transdermal innovations are fast arriving in the cannabis market, including long-lasting patches and tingly lubricants for medical patients and recreational consumers alike.

Strain-specific topicals attempt to

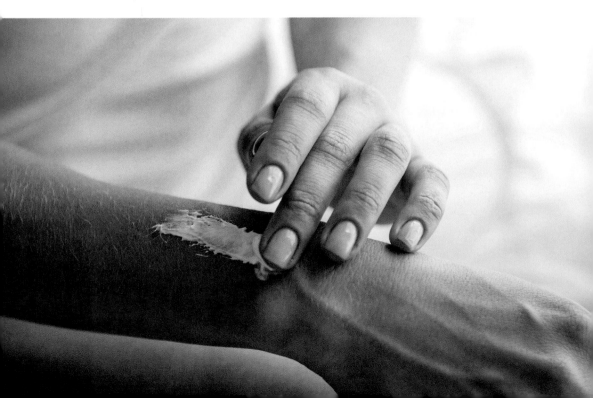

compile certain terpenes and cannabi-noids in a chemical profile similar to that of Blackberry Kush, Sour Diesel, or what-ever other strain the producer wishes to imitate. Along with THC, CBD, THCA, and other cannabinoids, topical producers may also select ingredients and essential oils for additional relief, like cayenne, wintergreen, and clove.

How Do Cannabis-Infused Topicals Work?

Cannabis-infused lotions, salves, oils, sprays, and other transdermal methods of relief work by binding to a network of receptors called CB2. These CB2 receptors are found throughout the body and are activated either by the body's naturally occurring endocannabinoids or by canna-bis compounds known as phytocannabi-noids (e.g., THC and CBD).

Even if a topical contains active THC, it still won't induce that intense "high" you'd get from smoking or ingesting can-nabis. With most topicals, cannabinoids can't breach the bloodstream; they only penetrate to the system of CB2 receptors. Transdermal patches, however, do deliver cannabinoids to the bloodstream and could have psychoactive effects with a high enough THC content.

What Symptoms Can Topicals Treat?

Topicals are most popularly chosen for localized pain relief, muscle soreness, tension, and inflammation, but anecdotal evidence is beginning to show a widen-ing spectrum of potential benefits, for the likes of psoriasis, dermatitis, itching, headaches, and cramping.

A THC-rich rub infused with cooling menthol and peppermint is a perfect way to wind down from a brutal work-out or hike. For intense localized pain, you may try a warming balm that com-bines the deep painkilling properties of cannabinoids with a tingling, soothing sensation. Inflammation symptoms may require a different chemical profile, as Cannabis Basics CEO Ah Warner explains: "Arthritic pain is caused by inflammation.

My products have [THCA] and CBD, both of which are anti-inflammatory. Active THC is not for inflammation, but when left in its acid form and combined with CBD, the two work to get rid of inflamma-tion and the pain that comes with it."

Different topicals offer different ben-efits depending on the way they are pro-cessed and the ingredients that are used, so experiment with various transdermal products to see what works for you. States with medical marijuana are seeing more and more options for topical remedies as time goes on, and for sufferers of pain and inflammation, they're worth explor-ing. You'd be surprised by the difference that one special ingredient makes.

Cannabis and Skin Care

WHETHER IT'S ACNE or eczema, treating troubled skin can feel like a battleground. There are a thousand things one can try, from over-the-counter creams and face washes to prescription ointments and pills. For some, there will be success with these methods—for others, however, the quest for clear and healthy skin can be ongoing and frustrating.

Fortunately, for those who have exhausted all conventional methods, or for those who desire a plant-based natural solution, cannabis may be your skin care answer.

Cannabis's Skin Care Potential

It's no surprise that cannabis may possess skin-healing benefits. All the elements are there. Cannabis is a known anti-inflammatory, with antioxidant and antiaging properties. In addition, hemp seed oil contains omega-3 and omega-6 fatty acids, which provide moisture and protection from sun damage.

The endocannabinoid system consists of many cannabinoid receptors, and a large portion of these are found in the skin. Molecules in cannabis such as THC

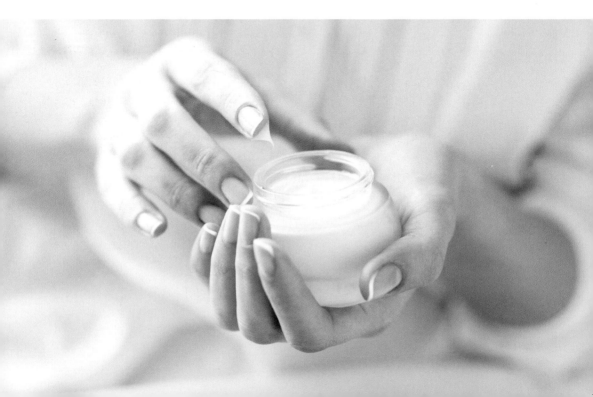

and CBD interact with this system to create the aforementioned positive effects.

Of course, when it comes to skin care, topicals are key. Smoke, no matter the substance, is never favorable to skin. In fact, if skin care is on the forefront of one's mind, it may be wise to forego smoking altogether in exchange for vaporizing or edibles. For targeted healing, there is a range of topical products to consider trying. Hemp oil and cannabis-derived CBD oil, for example, are gaining popularity as skin remedies.

Treating Skin Conditions with Cannabis

Study after study show the potential for cannabis to revolutionize the skin care world, and yet the topic remains rather obscure. Still, one need not look far to hear the stories of those who have been successful using cannabis for all types of skin ailments. Anecdotal evidence hints at the potential of CBD to cure contact dermatitis. Studies have shown potential benefits of cannabinoids in the treatment of psoriasis, due to its anti-inflammatory properties. Other accounts tout success using cannabis as a treatment for everything from acne to eczema.

When one considers how prevalent skin conditions are, it becomes clear that a safe, effective treatment is not only necessary but will be largely embraced by a huge subset of the population. The American Academy of Dermatology reports that fifty million Americans are affected by acne annually, and although the majority of sufferers are under the age of twenty-four, approximately 15 percent of those afflicted are older adults. Reported costs of treating acne are said to collectively exceed $3 billion.

And that's just acne alone. Combine those statistics with the approximately 7.5 million U.S. citizens who have psoriasis, 28 million who have (specifically) atopic dermatitis, and the billion-dollar anti-aging market, and a very clear picture is painted. Skin care remedies are a deeply sought after and much needed treatment. It says a lot that the market is so oversaturated with variations of creams, pills, and washes, both prescription and non-prescription. Some will find relief in variations of these products. For others, the search for relief seems endless. In truth, there has been no single guaranteed solution, no matter what the flashy commercials may have one believe.

However, as studies on the effects of cannabis skin care continue to emerge, and the understanding of the endo-cannabinoid system and its receptors improves, a new, unprecedented skin care market may well begin to develop. Although it will surely include a range of products like its predecessor, with mixed creams and balms containing all manner of oils in conjunction with cannabis, the beauty of cannabis skin care is that when all is said and done, the main ingredient, whether it be CBD, THC, or a combination thereof, will be readily available to make as luxurious or as simple of a treatment as desired.

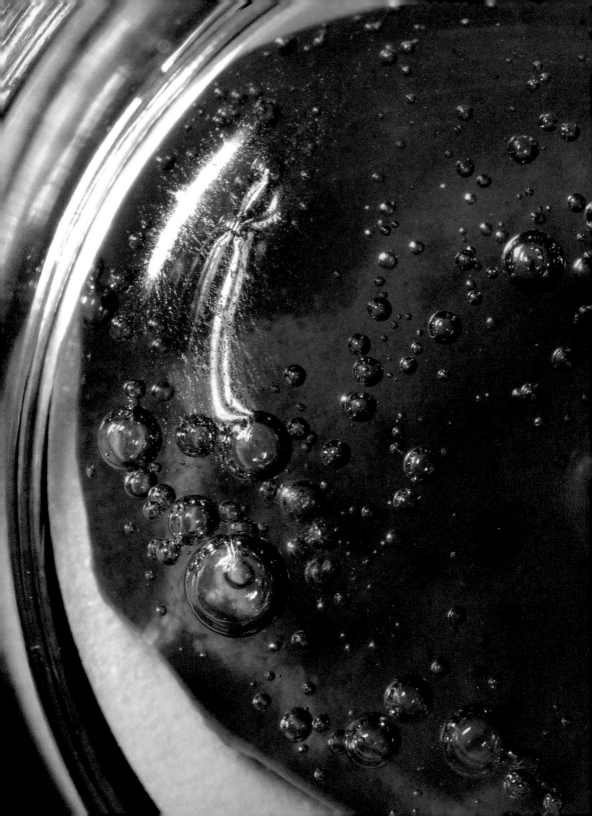

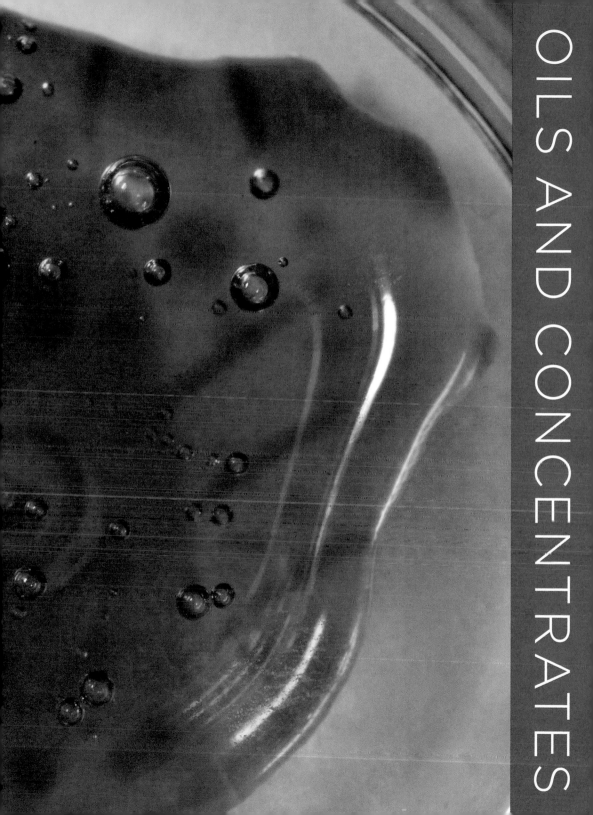

OILS AND CONCENTRATES

What Is a Cannabis Concentrate?

"CONCENTRATE" IS BECOMING an increasingly vague word in the cannabis industry. It could refer to the wax you vaporize, the tincture under your tongue, or the orally administered THC-free cannabis oil that's changing attitudes toward cannabis everywhere. The future of cannabis is steering toward these potent concentrated forms, especially as the therapeutic potential of nonsmoking methods is realized by the public.

Under the umbrella of cannabis concentrates falls any product procured through an extraction process. Solvents (e.g., butane, CO_2, ethanol) strip compounds from the cannabis plant, leaving behind a product with cannabinoids packed in every drop. Some types of extracts test as high as 80 percent in THC, while others are rich in nonpsychoactive compounds like CBD and deliver an altogether "high-less" experience.

This list of cannabis concentrates is by no means exhaustive, but it will introduce you to some of the most common extracts found in today's legal cannabis market.

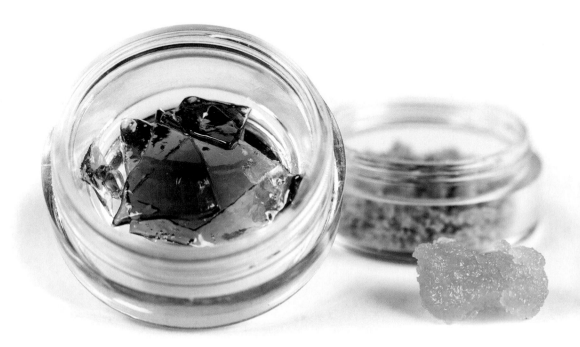

Hash

One of the oldest players in the cannabis game is hash, a concentrate made by compression of the plant's resin. The powdery kief that coats your cannabis flowers can be collected and pressed together to form hash, or solvents like ice water or ethanol may be used to more effectively strip the plant of their cannabinoid-loaded crystals. Though not as potent as BHO (see below) and other cannabis concentrates, hash remains a staple of cannabis culture around the world.

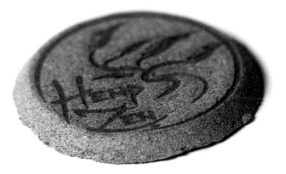

HASH HISTORY

The word "hashish" originates from the Arabic language, roughly translating to mean "grass." It is believed that the popularization of hash originated around AD 900, although some argue methods such as "charas," or the collection of resin from the hands of cannabis farmers, are believed to have existed prior to written documentation.

Butane Hash Oil (BHO)

BHO, or butane hash oil, is an extremely potent concentrate popularly consumed via dabbing and other vaporization methods. Cannabinoids are drawn out of the

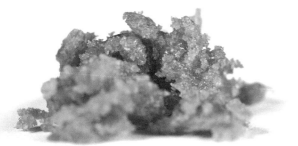

plant through butane extraction, which leaves behind a substance that will either maintain its sticky consistency or harden up, resulting in a syrupy oil, crumbly "wax," or a glasslike "shatter." Because its THC content stretches up to 80 percent, BHO is a popular remedy for chronic pain and other intractable symptoms. Always be sure that your oil is lab-tested for purity, as improperly purged BHO may contain traces of butane.

CO2 Oil

Hot on the market is CO2 oil, a concentrate made possible by expensive botanical extractors that use pressure and carbon dioxide to separate out plant material. This method, called supercritical fluid extraction, is one of the most effective ways of reducing cannabis to its essential compounds. The amber oil it produces can be vaporized in a variety of ways, one of the most popular being portable vaporizer pens. Among the industry's best sellers are disposable cartridges containing CO2 oil and a medical-grade solvent called polypropylene glycol, which gives the oil its liquid consistency.

Rosin

Rosin refers to an extraction process that utilizes a combination of heat and pressure to nearly instantaneously squeeze resinous sap from your initial starting material. The term "rosin" originated from the product used to lubricate violin bows. With cannabis, this method is incredibly versatile in that it can either be used with flowers or to clean up hash and kief into a full-melt hash oil. The result is a translucent, sappy, and sometimes shatterlike product.

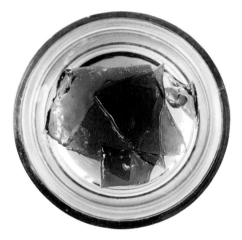

RICK SIMPSON OIL (RSO)

In 2003 a man named Rick Simpson treated his skin cancer using a homemade remedy made from cannabis. By soaking the cannabis in pure naphtha or isopropyl alcohol, the therapeutic compounds are drawn out of the plant, leaving behind a tarlike liquid after the solvent fully evaporates. Rick Simpson Oil (RSO) can be orally administered or applied directly to the skin. Many other businesses now sell their own renditions of RSO, some of which are high in THC while others contain only nonpsychoactive compounds like CBD.

Tinctures

Up until its prohibition in 1937, tinctures were the most common form of cannabis medicine in the United States. A tincture is a liquid concentrate procured through alcohol extraction, which pulls out many of the plant's beneficial cannabinoids. A few drops under the tongue may be a sufficient dose, but patients can safely apply more as needed. Tinctures, which are now available in a variety of flavors, are a great way for patients to medicate without having to smoke.

What's the Difference between Cannabis Oil, Shatter, and Wax?

Shatter, wax, honeycomb, oil, crumble, sap, budder, pull-and-snap . . . these are some of the descriptive nicknames cannabis extracts have earned through their popularity, prevalence, and diversification. If you've heard any of those words before, they were likely used to describe BHO (butane hash oil), CO2 oil, or similar hydrocarbon extracts. But what's the difference between oil, shatter, and wax? You may find that in the end, they're not so different after all.

"Cannabis oil" is a generalized term used to describe shatter, wax, RSO, and many other types of cannabis extracts. For now, we're going to jump into the two most common types of oils used for dabbing: shatter and wax, two extracts whose differences are pretty superficial.

WHAT IS SHATTER?

Shatter, with its flawless amber-colored glasslike transparency, has a reputation for being the purest and cleanest type of extract. But translucence isn't necessarily the telltale sign of quality—the consistency and texture of oil comes down to different factors entirely.

The reason shatter comes out perfectly clear has to do with the molecules that, if left undisturbed, form a glasslike appearance. Heat, moisture, and high terpene contents can also affect the texture, turning oils into a runnier substance that resembles syrup (hence the nickname "sap"). Oil with a consistency that falls somewhere between glassy shatter and viscous sap is often referred to as "pull-and-snap."

WHAT IS WAX?

Cannabis wax refers to the softer, opaque oils that have lost their transparency after extraction. Unlike those of transparent oils, the molecules of cannabis wax crystallize as a result of agitation. Light can't travel through irregular molecular densities, and that refraction leaves us with a solid, nontransparent oil.

Just as transparent oils span the spectrum between shatter and sap, wax can also take on different consistencies based on heat, moisture, and the texture of the oil before it is purged (the process in which residual solvents are removed from the product). Runny oils with more moisture tend to form gooey waxes ("budder"), while the harder ones are likely to take on a soft, brittle texture known as crumble or honeycomb. The term "wax" can be used to describe all of these softer, solid textures.

What Is Dabbing and What Are the Risks and Benefits?

IF YOU'VE PAID any attention to the world of cannabis as it's legalized in many states across the United States, then you probably know about or have heard of "dabbing." Dabbing as a method of consumption has been around for at least a decade, but the advent of more advanced extraction methods has led to a flood of cannabis concentrates that have boosted dabbing's popularity.

A dab refers to a dose of concentrate that is heated on a hot surface, usually a nail, and then inhaled through a dab rig. It doesn't sound so controversial in those terms, but "blasting dabs" has become a dividing point within the community both because of the intense high that it produces and for the image that it presents to outsiders.

While there are valid concerns to be

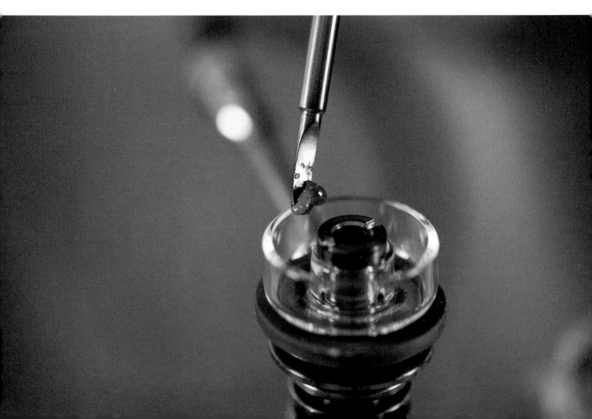

addressed about the safety of the production and potency of popular concentrates, this new trend isn't all bad. Here's the breakdown on the issues surrounding dabs and how it might actually be a good thing for the legalization movement.

What Are Dabs and How Are They Made?

Dabs are concentrated doses of cannabis that are made by extracting THC and other cannabinoids using a solvent like butane or carbon dioxide, resulting in sticky oils also commonly referred to as wax, shatter, budder, and butane hash oil (BHO) (see our previous chapter on concentrates for more). While it's possible to extract nonpsychoactive compounds like CBD, THC is what's behind the potent effects of dabs, making them the fastest and most efficient way to get really, really stoned. Terpenes, or the aromatic oils that give cannabis flavor, can also be extracted, although it can be difficult to preserve these volatile compounds in the extraction process.

What Are the Risks Associated with Dabbing?

Let's start with what many of you may have already heard: In certain groups, dabbing has a bad reputation. It's important to separate the myths and the facts by separating out two key parts of dabbing: the manufacturing of the cannabis concentrate that people are going to consume in their dab rig, and the act of consumption itself.

Any kind of home extraction can be dangerous, can lead to a poor product, and is not recommended. Thanks to online forums and videos, many amateur "scientists" think they have mastered the technique of cannabis extraction enough to try it on their own. In cases when things go well, the product is probably still pretty poor. When things go bad, houses can blow up.

Another side effect of these home extraction experiments is "dirty" oil that may contain chemical contaminants that could present health hazards to consumers.

If the concern is butane, the dangers may be minimal since it already occurs in everyday products such as scent and flavor extracts. Whether or not the equipment used in the extraction process is adding additional contaminants is a more reasonable issue. When done correctly, these extras can be avoided, so as is the case with

Torch-less Dabbing

Not all dabbing apparatuses require the use of a torch. E-nails, for example, plug into an outlet and heat to whatever temperature you set them to. Low-temperature dabbing is a better dabbing method to make the most of your oil's terpenes. New dabbing technology is also emerging, offering the full dabbing experience without the dangers associated with a torch and hot nail.

growing cannabis, it's best to leave it to those who know what they're doing.

Additionally, the actual process of dabbing can look quite scary. Glass bongs and oddly named substances being heated with blowtorches have led to the comparison that dabs are the "crack" of pot. It's not that BHO has any similarity to these harsher drugs, but to the uninitiated, lighting something with a torch looks unsafe and may carry safety risks.

One of the most unsettling facts about dabs is that thanks to the superconcentrated power of BHO, it seems possible to "overdose" on cannabis. Taking more than your personal limit of dabs can lead to a bad experience and, in some cases, feeling ill and passing out. After all the chanting that "you can't overdose on cannabis," concentrates could be undermining advocates' message of safety. There have also been reports of more intense withdrawal symptoms for dabbers, but again, the information is limited. Regardless, while whether or not to dab is a matter of choice for most consumers, there are fears that dabbing's ugly looks and home extraction risks may hurt the legalization movement.

MYTH: DABBING IS ALL ABOUT THC

Dabbing doesn't necessarily have to be about getting as high as humanly possible. High-CBD dabs may work for the anxiety prone or patients needing a swift dose of relief. Pay attention to terpene content, too. Terpenes are often lost in the extraction process, but devoted producers will take extra care in preserving or reintroducing terpenes to create a more nuanced and pleasant dabbing experience.

Are There Medical Benefits to Dabbing?

The biggest positive of concentrates are that they can give a powerful dose of relief to those who truly need it. Patients dealing with severe or chronic pain or extreme nausea report that dabbing can be one of the best ways to get immediate and effective relief. The amount of flower that would have to be smoked or vaporized to get the same effect is just unfeasible for some patients who need potent relief quickly.

Yes, the safety issues associated with making extracts are real, but they can be minimized in a professional environment. Professional extractors eschew the dangerous "open" extraction method that can (but should not) be done at home and instead choose closed extraction, which is safer but requires more sophisticated equipment and knowledge. Also, there are other extraction methods, such as CO_2 or ice-water extraction, that are safer and reduce or remove the possibility of explosions.

The relationship between concentrates and technology is at a compelling moment: This is a product greatly in need of more research, and an industry which requires high levels of testing. Because the legal marketplace is expanding and more and more producers are improving and upgrading their methods, it seems likely that these homemade disasters should become anomalies. Technology is also probably going to lead to less dabbing in the future, anyway. Improvements in vaporizers mean that more people are using these "no-torch necessary" products to heat their oils. Conveniently, this is the most publicity-friendly path for concentrates to go.

While dabbing may be going through its awkward phase, overall, concentrates have much to offer patients and legal cannabis consumers in the future, and dabs are just one option among many.

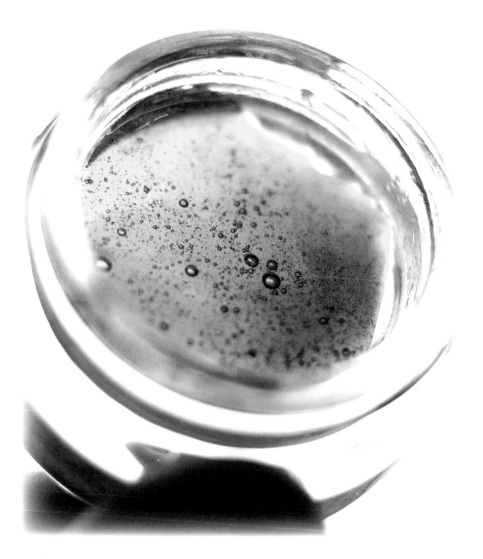

How to Dab Cannabis Concentrates

DABBING ISN'T FOR everyone, especially if you're new to cannabis entirely, inexperienced in the method, or in an unsafe environment. The dosing process is more delicate and requires greater attention to safety, so if it's your first time, you're probably best off experiencing it with someone who's been there and done that before.

But if you've gotten the hang of it, concentrates may offer you new heights of physical relief and unique cerebral effects. Extracts also contain a lot less plant material than flower, so you're inhaling more cannabinoids (e.g., THC, CBD) and less combusted resin.

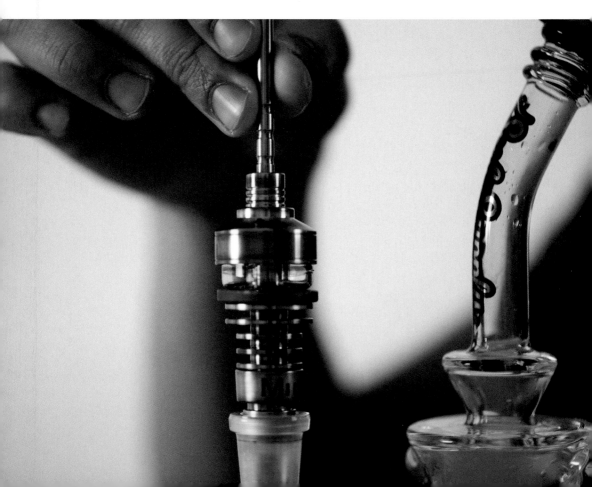

Tools You'll Need to Dab

Dabbing technology is evolving, but the traditional setup includes the following items (keep in mind that the appearance of each tool may vary slightly depending on its design):

1. *A cannabis extract.* These come in a variety of forms, but the most common ones used for dabbing are BHO, CO_2, and solvent-less extracts like rosin.

2. *A water pipe.* You can take the glass bowl pieces out and replace them with dabbing attachments to turn your pipe into a dab rig.

3. *A nail.* Find a nail that fits your water pipe's gauge. Some are made of ceramic and quartz, but titanium is the most commonly used type.

4. *A dome.* This is the glass hood placed around the nail. "Dome-less" nails don't need one, but standard nails need something to trap the vapor before it's inhaled.

5. *A torch.* Culinary torches used for crème brûlée will do the job, but some choose to upgrade to larger propane-fueled torches that heat nails faster. New flameless methods of dabbing are becoming available, but the less-safe torch method is still most popular due to the low cost.

6. *A dabber.* This is the glass, metal, or ceramic tool used to apply a dab.

How to Dose a Dab

Different extracts have different THC concentrations, so it's helpful to know how potent your oil is before dabbing with it. However, it's generally recommended to start small and increase the dose if you feel comfortable doing so.

A small dose is no bigger than a crumb. It may not look like much, but that's still a lot of THC going straight to the dome at once. Dabbing can feel more intense to those accustomed to flower, but as your tolerance adjusts, the effects become less jarring.

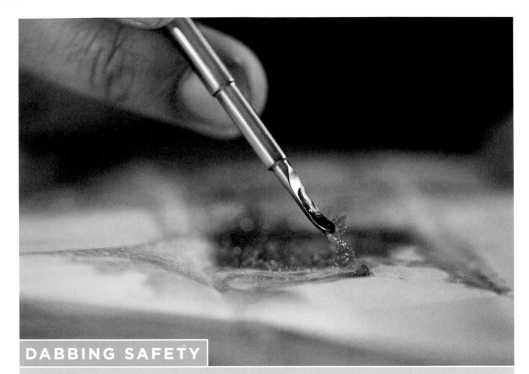

DABBING SAFETY

1. Always be very, very careful when handling the torch, taking care never to drop it or knock it over to avoid burning yourself. Make sure the knob is turned all the way off when you're finished, so butane gas does not leak out.

2. Make sure the nail isn't red hot when applying your dab. This temperature is too hot, so let the nail cool for 10 to 15 seconds to avoid burning your throat with the inhale.

3. Taking dabs in a seated position may help prevent feelings of light-headedness.

4. Hydrate, hydrate, hydrate. Water may help prevent some of the unpleasant side effects of THC.

5. Make sure your concentrate has been tested for residual solvents to ensure purity.

Disclaimer: Dabbing, like other methods of consumption, is done at your own risk and should only be done in legal states. It raises safety concerns. Take caution when handling the torch and other necessary tools, and wait for all pieces to cool before handling.

How to Take a Dab

Once the rig is set up and your dab is prepared on the dabber, you're ready to get started. We advise you to sit while taking a dab, since the rush of THC can be physically intense.

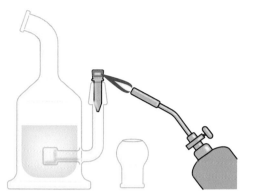

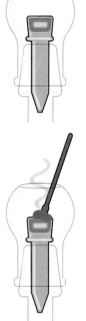

Step 1:

Turn on your torch and aim the flame directly at the nail. Some people will heat the nail until it begins to turn red hot.

Note: Nails and glass domes become extremely hot in the dabbing process. Take caution when handling them, and always wait for all pieces to cool down completely before you even think of touching them.

Step 2:

Once the nail is hot, turn off your torch and place the glass dome over the nail. It's recommended to let titanium nails cool for about 10 seconds and quartz nails about 45 seconds so the surface temperature isn't too hot.

Step 3:

Take your dabber, apply the dab directly on the nail inside the dome, and inhale slowly. Rotating the dabber tip on the nail can help you prevent wasting any oil stuck to the dabber.

Step 4:

Exhale and enjoy!

What Is Rosin and How Can I Make It at Home?

ROSIN USES A solvent-less extraction technique that allows anybody to make their own high-quality hash oil from the comfort of their home. Aesthetically, rosin is almost impossible to distinguish from shatter or sap. However, the difference between the two is that rosin is completely free of the residual solvents often left behind by hydrocarbon extraction processes (e.g., butane, propane), and therefore free of the risks that go with those other forms of at-home extraction.

Rosin can be made safely and inexpensively in just minutes by using ordinary household tools. This method utilizes heat and pressure to squeeze the cannabinoid-rich resin from your flowers, bubble hash, or kief. Your average hair straightener, some parchment paper, and a collection tool are all that's needed to produce a hash oil that rivals hydrocarbon extraction methods in flavor, potency, and effect.

Rosin is certainly making an impact in the legal cannabis market. Dispensaries all over the country are beginning to stock their shelves with this easily crafted, incredibly potent, and flavorful product. Let's find out how it can be made.

Ingredients Needed to Make Rosin at Home

1. Hair straightener (try to find one with a temperature setting of around 300°F or lower—any higher and you begin to lose valuable terpenes as they evaporate)

2. Cannabis (this can be flower, bubble hash, or kief)

3. Parchment paper (unbleached, if possible)

4. Collection tool (many dabber tools work well here, although you can get creative!)

5. Heat-resistant gloves for safety

> **Note:** Like other methods, this is done at your own risk. Please exercise caution when handling the hair straightener and use heat-resistant gloves as an added safety measure—we don't want you to burn yourself!

Four Simple Steps to Make Rosin

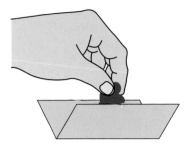

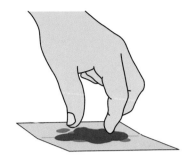

Step 1:

Turn on your hair straightener to the lowest setting (280°F to 330°F) and cut yourself a small 4 × 4-inch piece of parchment paper. Now fold it in half and place your cannabis material in between the folded parchment paper before giving it a light preliminary finger press.

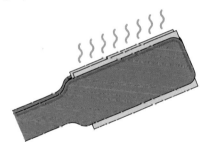

Step 3:

Remove your sample from the hot surface and unfold the parchment paper. Now pluck the flattened nug away and grab your collection tool. This is a very sticky process so be patient and careful. For larger batches, use different clean sheets of parchment and collect your samples together at the end.

Step 2:

Carefully line the buds inside of the paper together with your hair straightener and apply a very firm pressure for 3 to 7 seconds. You will want to hear a sizzle before you release the pressure—it indicates that the resin has melted from the plant material.

Step 4 (Optional):

Remove any visible plant material if you wish. Fold the finished product between the parchment and flatten it to your preference. Then use a clean tool to pick out any plant particulates. You may place the substance on a cold surface for a few seconds if you desire a more stable material to work with.

Now load a nice fat dab of your fresh new rosin and celebrate! You just became an extract artist!

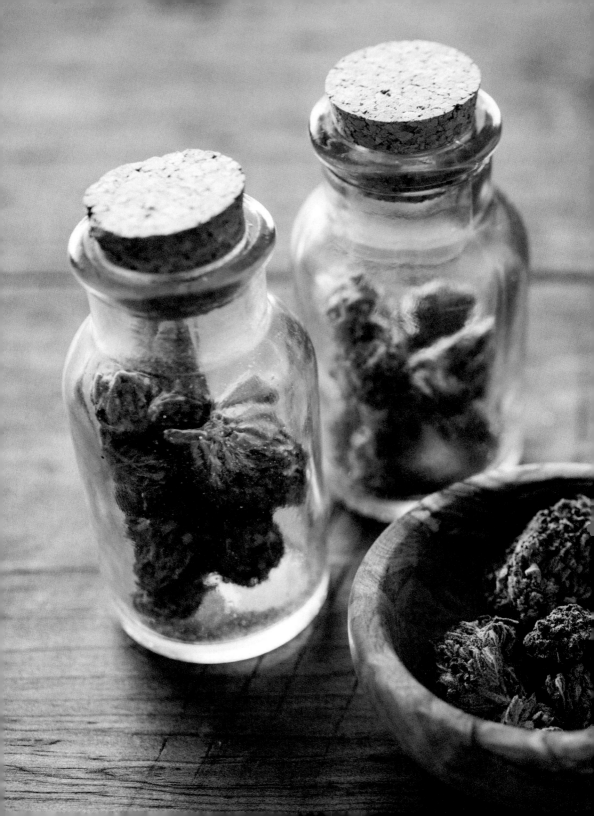

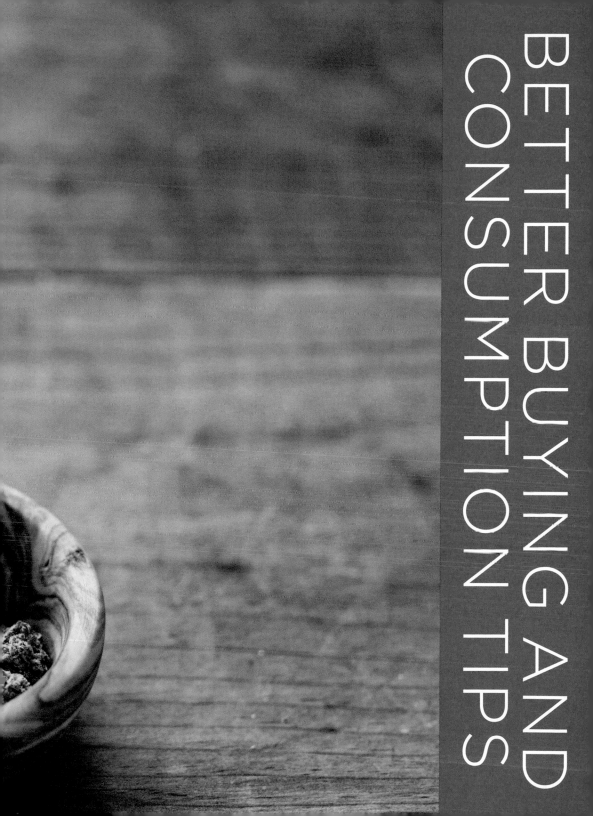

BETTER BUYING AND CONSUMPTION TIPS

What to Expect on Your First Dispensary Visit

ALTHOUGH DISPENSARIES MAY be legal in your state now, it can still feel intimidating to visit one for the first time and not know what to do, which questions to ask, or how to find the products you want. Whether you're planning to visit a retail cannabis shop or a medical marijuana dispensary, if you familiarize yourself with these basic guidelines, you'll feel more comfortable with the process and can better focus your efforts on finding the products you want.

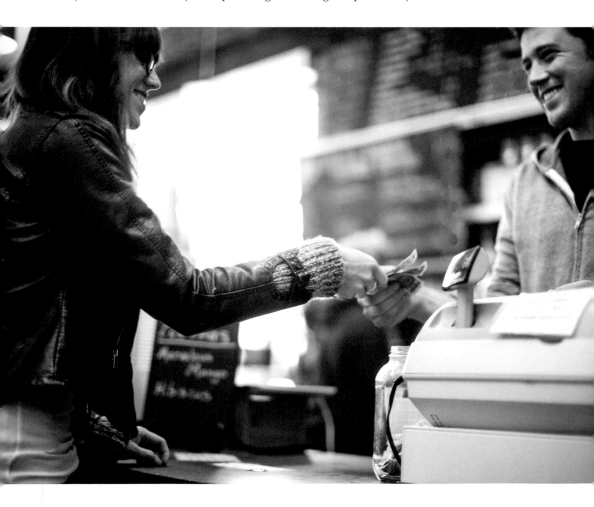

Bring Your State-Issued ID

Whether you're an adult consumer or a medical marijuana patient, expect to get carded as soon as you enter the dispensary. Even if you end up becoming a return visitor or a regular customer, bring your state-issued identification with you every time and be prepared to show it to both security personnel and the budtender helping you. Dispensaries must remain in strict compliance with state laws, and if they get caught being lax on the rules or selling to minors, they could undermine their state's legal cannabis program as well as the legalization movement growing across the country.

Have a Copy of Your Medical Marijuana Recommendation (If Applicable)

If you're a new medical marijuana patient, the dispensary will need to verify your doctor's recommendation before you're legally allowed to purchase anything. Bring your authorization with you so the dispensary can make a copy of it and keep it on file. Some dispensaries are able to accept your doctor's recommendation as an email attachment before you visit their location, or you can call the dispensary ahead of time and provide your doctor's contact information so they can follow up with your doctor and verify the authorization. Whatever the dispensary's process, understand that you need to follow its protocol so that your state's program can continue to run smoothly and legally.

Find a Preferred Dispensary

You'll want to find a dispensary that you're comfortable visiting. Dispensaries range in caliber, style, and selection, so make sure you're informed before you go. It's worth trying a few out in your local area to see what fits the kind of experience you're looking for.*

* Among available resources, Leafly's dispensary finder can help you choose a location that's convenient, browse menus on dispensary pages, and its strain or product finder can help locate a dispensary or store that carries a particular strain or product.

Be Prepared to Wait

In many states, regulations require dispensaries to serve only one patient at a time, so you may need to take a seat and wait your turn. Use this time to look through the dispensary's menu and think about what strains or products you'd like.

Ask Questions

Whether you know what you want ahead of time or aren't sure which strains to try, one of the best ways to get your bearings during a dispensary visit is to ask your budtender for advice. Get recommendations on strains they like, or ask for strains that might be best suited for your needs. Let the budtender be your guide. Looking for something to settle your stomach? Ask. Want a bright sativa to inspire you to finally deep-clean your house? Ask. Budtenders are accustomed to helping new and inexperienced customers, so remember that there are no stupid questions.

Bring Cash for Your Purchase

Most cannabis shops are forced to be cash-only due to federal restrictions on banking. Some dispensaries and retail shops offer cashless ATM systems, but before you visit a new location, check to see whether they accept debit cards or have an ATM onsite. Otherwise, be prepared and bring cash to make your purchase go as smoothly as possible.

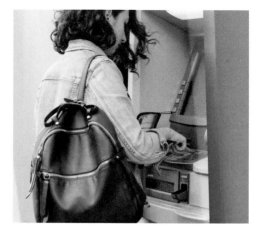

Don't Feel Pressured or Uncomfortable

If something about the dispensary is making you uncomfortable (such as the employees, decor, or product quality), you're under no obligation to stay and make a purchase. Remember, in most cases, returns are forbidden by law, so once you buy a strain or product, it's yours (provided there's no recall or other outstanding issue). If the dispensary doesn't have what you want in stock or its budtenders aren't being helpful or are pushing products you're not interested in, you're free to say "no thank you" and leave to find a location that better suits you.

What Makes a Good Budtender?

WALKING INTO A dispensary and purchasing legal cannabis for the first time is both a wonderful and surreal experience. Customers find themselves immersed in a whole new world of strain varieties, extracts, edibles, topicals, and a myriad of other innovative products. In most cases, helping customers make their selections are budtenders, staff trained to help people find the products that will best suit their needs.

Unfortunately, not all budtenders are created equal. In fact, their competency and helpfulness can vary drastically depending on a number of variables. Be on the lookout for the following positive traits exhibited by good budtenders—they'll offer a strong indication that your dispensary experience will be a positive one.

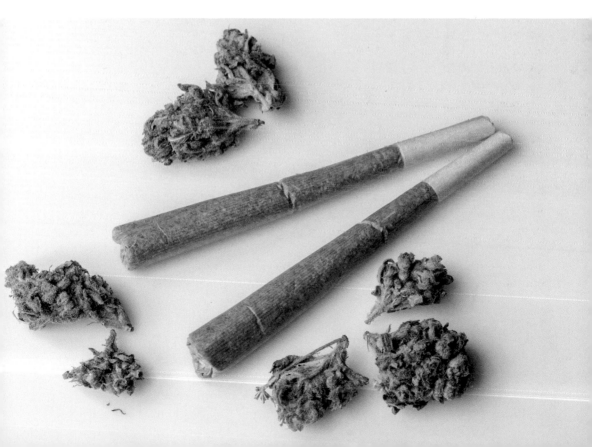

They Know the Product Well and Handle It Respectfully

Successful budtenders know the store's inventory and can speak to the different nuances within each product and strain.

When showing the bud or product to customers, budtenders are clean and avoid touching product with bare hands.

They Create Relationships with Their Customers

Despite the constant influx of customers throughout the day, good budtenders remember their regulars and are able to suggest new products based on their previous purchases. Or, at the very least, they go out of their way to have a positive interaction with customers and visitors and work to understand why they walked through the door in order to make recommendations based on their needs.

They're Passionate about Cannabis and Its Surrounding Culture

Not every customer or patient bleeds green, but many do seek a sense of culture and passion in the stores or dispensaries they frequent. Budtenders have the ability to deliver this element, making a customer's purchase more of an experience than an exchange.

Good budtenders know industry influencers, important cannabis holidays and events, and a solid amount of background information about cannabis to create that positive interaction with their patrons. Their passion and industry savviness help position them as a credible resource for cannabis information.

They Tailor Their Service to All Levels of Experience

Each customer has a unique relationship and experience with cannabis. Tailoring explanations to an individual's level of familiarity with cannabis sets the great budtenders apart from the rest of the crew. The best budtenders leave first-time consumers and veterans feeling the same way: happy, heard, and satisfied.

How to Help Your Budtender Recommend the Perfect Product for You

HELPFUL BUDTENDERS WILL typically ask more questions than they are asked themselves, allowing them to customize product recommendations. An adept budtender will not only know the specification of every product they sell, but can separate which products to recommend by asking questions and narrowing down options until they've found the ideal strain or consumable for their patron.

To help your budtender make better recommendations for you, ask yourself these five questions. These queries are no different from what an experienced budtender would ask you, so give some consideration to your answers in order to make your dispensary experience a successful one.

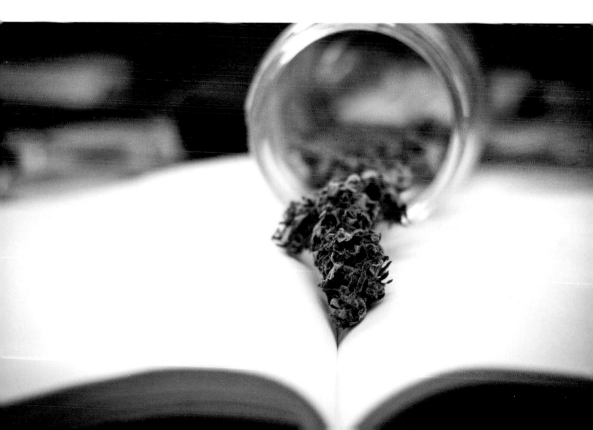

How Would You Like to Consume Your Cannabis?

Cannabis can be consumed in a myriad of different ways, from smoking flower to rubbing infused creams on sore muscles. Research which way you would like to consume cannabis, or arm yourself with a few questions about various consumption methods so that your budtender can help guide you along.

Are You Seeking Cannabis as Medicine?

If you plan to use cannabis medicinally, you may be interested in different strains and consumption methods than someone who uses it for personal wellness or enhancement purposes. Even if you're visiting a retail cannabis shop, you should first consult with a physician educated in medical marijuana so that you can explain what your symptoms are and see if they recommend a particular consumption method or strain. Remember, your budtender is not your doctor, so it's important to get a valid medical opinion before you ask your budtender for recommendations. That way, you can take both perspectives into account to better understand what type of relief you need.

How Psychoactive of an Experience Can You Tolerate?

Cannabis can affect your mental and physical state in vastly different ways depending on the product type, dosage, and consumption method. These variables change even more when factoring in your tolerance levels. Certain products may seem appealing but could be too intense for your liking. Others can be uplifting and cerebral when you're looking for something relaxing and sedating. Letting your budtender know what your tolerance levels are like and what experience you're seeking will help them guide you toward a product that will meet your exact needs.

How Long Do You Wish to Feel the Effects?

Planning out how you intend to use cannabis is important and will help in determining both the products and consumption methods you discuss with your budtender. For example, dabbing tends to provide a quick and intense experience when compared to edibles, while edibles take time to kick in but can have effects that last for hours, even days, depending on their potency. Whether you're looking for a quick onset with moderate effects or something that will take longer to kick in but provides intense relief, communicate your expectations to your budtender to narrow down your options.

How Discreet Must Your Cannabis Consumption Be?

Using cannabis discreetly can be a matter of courtesy. Cannabis smoke and vapor may bother some people. It's important to be considerate to others in all situations, but it's vital to understand how your cannabis use is going to affect those around y   u're planning to be in the pres-
          ers who choose not to consume cannabis, bring this to the attention of your budtender so that they can guide you toward products that can be used anywhere. Edibles, vape pens, topicals, sublinguals, transdermals, capsules, and even suppositories are examples of discreet products.

How to Find the Best Strain, Product, and Consumption Method for You

ACCESS TO LEGAL cannabis is now available to more people than ever before, and with that access come options and opportunity. Navigating the vast array of strains, products, and consumption methods legal markets are offering today can be a dizzying ordeal, as there isn't a "one size fits all" cannabis experience that's right for everyone.

Narrowing down the selection process can be the differentiating factor between an enjoyable cannabis experience and an overwhelming, negative interaction. Here are a few helpful hints to help you determine which strain, product, and consumption method may be ideal for you.

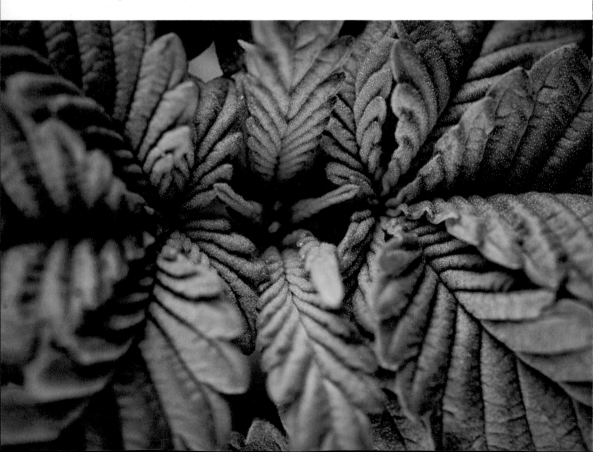

Ask Yourself a Few Questions

Before reaching out to anyone for help in personalizing your cannabis experience, ask yourself some preliminary questions as a vetting tool. This exercise will help to limit your options down to smaller groups of strains, products, and consumption methods.

- What is your experience level with cannabis? First-time users should most certainly consider this when choosing a means of consumption. For instance, dabbing a high-THC cannabis concentrate through a large rig is not a preferable consumption method for a beginner. Instead, newcomers may want to start off with small amounts of flower and/or a low-dose edible. If, however, you're experienced with cannabis and are looking for a more potent delivery option, concentrates may be a preferred method.

- Do you have a preference when it comes to things like combusted cannabis smoke or dietary restrictions? This consideration can impact what delivery method you choose. If you're worried about lung health or thick smoke odors, you may want to shy away from smoking cannabis via joints, bongs, or pipes, and instead opt for using vaporizers. If you're counting calories or have food allergies, edibles may be a more problematic consumption method than flower or topicals.

- Where will you be when enjoying this cannabis, and who will you be enjoying it with? If you plan on going out and about with lots of people and you know that you can enjoy a highly active sativa, vaporizer pens are a perfect fit. On the contrary, a night snuggled in solitude may better benefit from a relaxing edible or infused bath product. If you're sick, a tincture may be appealing. Need to be discreet? Infused candies, breath mints, and oral sprays work well.

Consult with a Local Budtender

Information in and of itself can be a labyrinth in disguise. There are thousands of distinct strain varietals indexed and numerous consumption options, as well as a burgeoning product marketplace churning out new technology by the minute. This makes personalizing an experience with cannabis more complex an endeavor than one may imagine. In fact, navigating your way through the options can feel like a full-time job.

And it is! Budtenders are your perfect allies when trying to narrow down the options. These industry professionals are there for one reason: to help you personalize your experience by eliminating the fear of the unknown. They're trained to ask you questions in order to guide you through the jungle of options out there.

Find a reputable dispensary in your area and pick your local budtender's brain with all of your cannabis-related questions.

There's nothing quite like a one-on-one experience with an industry professional if you're just starting out with cannabis. Their expertise is invaluable and an interpersonal dialogue with another human, even for just a few minutes, can often leave you with more information than an hour of searching the Internet.

Check In with a Head Shop

Not all dispensaries are equipped to offer you the exact product you're looking for when it comes to the plethora of cannabis delivery methods available, which is why building a relationship with the staff at your local head shop is so important.

What is a head shop? In simplest terms, a head shop is a place where you can go to find products that will help you consume your cannabis. In many places, head shops still advertise as a place to purchase tobacco-related products. Many tobacco "water pipe" retailers are incredibly knowledgeable and can help to answer your broader smoking-related questions just the same.

Head shop retailers can be an ir able asset in learning about deliv ods and getting set up with a pr suits your cannabis consumptio ences. Pipes, papers, vaporizers, g. s, you name it, they know about it.

With your quiver of resources bursting at the seams, finding help narrowing down options for an enjoyable cannabis experience should be a delightful undertaking. By arming yourself with the right questions and taking those considerations to your local professionals, choosing a strain, product, and delivery method is as simple as an afternoon out and about.

Recommended Strains and Products for Different Scenarios and Moods

CANNABIS IS UNIQUELY versatile in that it can be enjoyed in many different ways, offering a variety of experiences with each creative combination. Between the vast landscape of available strains, preparations, and products available, one could feasibly enjoy a different strain and consumption method for each individual scenario. Understanding this is important when discerning between conducive strains and activities. Just as there are many ways one may pair cannabis properly with a given situation, it can be just as easy to improperly pair cannabis, leaving you with a potentially uncomfortable scenario.

Creating a conducive pairing is a learned skill, so here are a few situations based on time of day, mood, and activity where we recommend some appropriate strain types and consumption methods. Here are a small handful of our favorite combinations to try out, whether you're using cannabis to wake up and motivate yourself or to relax and unwind. (Keep in mind that these are merely our favorites; if you have a preferred consumption method, you're free to substitute one of our recommendations with your tried-and-true delivery method.)

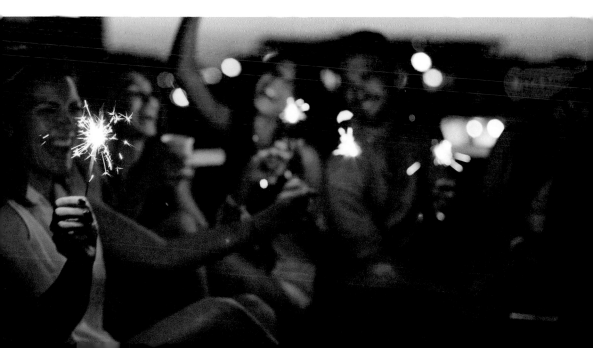

For Starting Out Your Day

Strain: A pure sativa (e.g., Durban Poison)

Medium: Concentrate or flower

Consumption method: Home vaporizer

Ideal for: A morning workout, running errands, tidying your space

Pure sativas like Durban Poison are essentially an espresso shot for the cannabis enthusiast. With the rise of hybridization, pure sativa strains are not easy to come by, but if your dispensaries carry them, pick up a strain or two as a morning pick-me-up. We enjoy pure sativas either by use of a flower or concentrate vaporizer before heading out. The energy this strain gives will complement any workout or morning activity perfectly!

After a Long Day

Strain: A hybrid (e.g., Fire OG)

Medium: Flower

Consumption method: Large tabletop water pipe

Ideal for: Unwinding with some relaxation time

Hybrids are often the preferred strain type for individuals looking for a relaxing solo couch session. Larger water pipes offer a "one hitter quitter," meaning you can feel the effects after one or two big hits. Fire OG is especially known for encouraging heavy relaxation without being too sleepy in the head rush, offering a perfect pairing for a night in with a favorite movie or TV show.

For Experimenting in the Kitchen

Strain: Any hybrid variety

Medium: Infused cooking oil

Consumption method: Edible

Ideal for: A dinner party with friends

Hybrid strains make for wonderful companions when it comes to infusing cooking oils for edibles. The next time a weekend dinner party is on the calendar, try infusing a hybrid strain into olive oil to be used for meal preparations. Infused oils are also available in some markets, so don't hesitate to ask your budtender about them.

When having guests over, it's important to consider the individual dosage preferences of each member in the party, which is why olive oil is a great infusion option. In this case, it can be offered as a tabletop condiment, such as an infused salad dressing, to be dosed to meet everyone's individual tolerances.

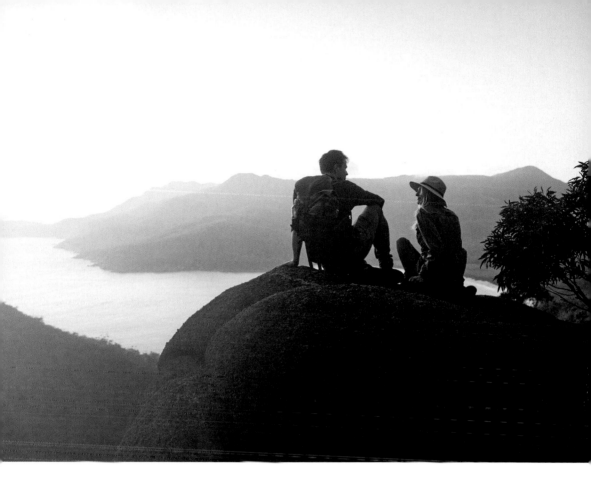

For Calm Self-Reflection

Strain: A high-CBD, indica-dominant option (e.g., Critical Mass)

Medium: Flower

Consumption method: Rolled joint

Ideal for: A peaceful walk

If one is in need of a stress-suppressing long walk, a mild indica-dominant hybrid like Critical Mass is a perfect companion.

Many phenotypes of this strain exhibit elevated levels of the known stress-reducing compound cannabidiol (CBD). Who doesn't like a nice joint and a peaceful walk? (Just make sure to enjoy cannabis in the most legal and noninvasive way possible when in populated spaces; also, keep in mind that many legal markets prohibit public consumption under penalty of fine or citation.)

For Discreet Consumption

Strain: Sativa-dominant hybrid (e.g., Sour Diesel)

Medium: CO_2 concentrate

Consumption method: Portable vaporizer pen

Ideal for: Quiet consumption while out and about

Unlike a joint, which can be rather odiferous when consumed in the presence of others, vaporizer pens loaded with CO_2 concentrates make for a discreet companion while you are out of the house (in a legal market, of course). A Sour Diesel extract, being a sativa-dominant hybrid, affords you the adequate energy boost you will need without alerting the world to your activities. Loaded in a vaporizer pen, this oil will last throughout your day while remaining as inconspicuous as it is portable.

For Relaxed Nonsmokers

Strain: Any indica-dominant variety

Medium: CBD-infused bath product

Consumption method: Topical application

Ideal for: Destressing after a long day

If inhalation causes coughing or other issues, certain strains make for fantastic infused products. Try a relaxing bubble bath with a CBD-infused bath bomb or topical lotion. These products are created by infusing cannabis concentrates into soaps and lotions for the purpose of topical applications. All cannabinoids, including THC and CBD, can be absorbed efficiently though the skin with a proper carrier oil.

For Late-Night Moments

Strain: A pure indica (e.g., Hindu Kush)

Medium: Concentrate

Consumption method: Tabletop dab rig (keeping in mind safety considerations; we don't want a burn at bedtime!)

Ideal for: A potent good night's sleep

Who needs a sleeping pill when there's a dab rig loaded with a pure indica concentrate around? Forget couch-lock; when dabbed out of a tabletop rig, indicas like Hindu Kush will send the consumer into a deep sleep. A strain like Hindu Kush is perfect for those "hard to fall asleep" occasions. Very rarely will a comfortable-size dab of a heavy indica concentrate leave you anywhere but in the folds of your pillow.

How to Pick the Best Quality Cannabis

PICKING OUT QUALITY cannabis is a lot like selecting fresh produce or flowers—you're looking for something that looks appealing, has a good color, and produces an enticing aroma. Cannabis buds have a number of visual cues that can help you determine their quality, and bad buds are pretty easy to spot if you know what to look for.

Before you begin to assess the visual quality of your cannabis, keep these key points in mind:

- Remember that quality standards may vary based on your location and access to cannabis, your personal experiences with the plant, and local cannabis laws (which must be complied with).

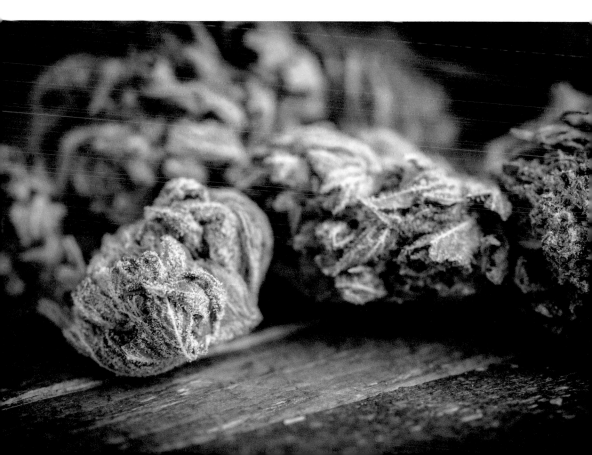

- There are many other attributes to consider when choosing the best strain for you, including the price, the smell, desired effects, and quantity available.

- A high concentration of trichomes on a bud indicates advanced cannabinoid production, which typically signifies potent cannabis. However, potent cannabis is not necessarily indicative of high quality—the strain could be lacking the flavor profile you're looking for, or, for example, it may be a stimulating sativa when you prefer a mellow indica.

- Test data can go a long way in visualizing and understanding the various attributes of each strain, so look for current and accurate test results from a trusted third-party laboratory if possible.

- Avoid any glaring defects like mold and mildew, insects, and discoloration.

Let's check out some examples of low, medium, and high-quality cannabis so you can better assess the quality of the buds you're acquiring.

Low-Quality Cannabis Buds

Also called: shwag, shake, bottom shelf, popcorn, dirt weed, brick weed, ditch weed, Bobby Brown

Effects: mellow, relaxing, lazy, and sleep-inducing due to the presence of the cannabinoid CBN; it's not uncommon to experience headaches and other adverse side effects from poorly grown and cared-for cannabis

Low-quality cannabis is often transported as compact bricks, resulting in a mix of shake, stems, and compressed buds. Shwag, which is rarely found in legal markets, tends to be less colorful than your average cannabis, often more brown than green (thus the nickname "Bobby Brown"—no relation to the former member of New Edition). It is dry and earthy in aroma with a taste that can be harsh and spicy, as opposed to the sweet and floral notes of top-grade cannabis. When they're

not compacted into brick weed, low-quality buds tend to be light, leafy, and wispy.

The concentration of cannabinoids is likely to be very low due to extreme environmental factors, like excessive heat or other variables that cause trichomes and other crucial parts of the plant to underdevelop. Harsh growing conditions are typical for low-quality, improperly cared-for cannabis and it has a tendency to be

> The cannabinoid known as cannabinol (or CBN) is a product of THC degradation. As THC oxidizes, it converts to CBN, a process that can be prompted by either heat or oxygen. Aged, poorly stored cannabis can have higher levels of CBN than fresh flower in an airtight container. CBN's strongest attribute is its sedating effect, with 5 milligrams of CBN as effective as 10 milligrams of diazepam, a mild pharmaceutical sedative.

high in the cannabinoid CBN, a by-product of degradation. Advanced levels of CBN are often attributed to poor or improper storage and handling during transportation.

One glaring advantage of low-quality cannabis is that it is usually available at discounted prices. Some cannabis consumers prefer to bargain hunt and turn their shwag into affordable cannabis-infused edibles.

Medium-Quality Cannabis Buds

Also called: mids, middle shelf, regs, Reggie, beasters, B+, work

Effects: can vary across the board, but generally if the genetics are strong, the resulting effects are potent and enjoyable

Medium-quality cannabis is where most domestically grown U.S. cannabis lands on the quality scale. Northern states also see an influx of mids and regs from commercial Canadian cannabis, known as beasters or BC buds (though the influx is starting to dwindle now that the United States is shifting toward legal access).

Mids can be identified by their spectrum of green hues and the presence of colorful pistils. Solid middle-shelf genetics showcase purple tinge, moderate flavor profiles, and sugary trichomes. Seeds and stems are minimal to none, but the buds can suffer from a number of quick-to-market techniques like improper flushing of nutrients, quick curing methods, and sloppy trim jobs. Pricing for middle quality is somewhat standardized based on your region, and oftentimes bulk discounts become available when buying more than a quarter or half ounce at a time.

Understanding Different Cannabis Quantities: A Visual Guide

Gram, eighth, ounce—what does it all mean? Attempting to make sense of the many different cannabis quantities can be challenging for newcomers. If you're heading to a dispensary for the first time and want to brush up on size differences before you go shopping, this helpful visual guide provides a general framework to better understand the common sale quantities for both flower and concentrates.

NOTE: Keep in mind that these depictions are approximations, given that density varies (at times drastically) between products.

Number of grams in an ounce:

⅛ ounce = 3.5 grams

¼ ounce = 7 grams

½ ounce = 14 grams

1 ounce = 28.35 grams

High-Quality Cannabis Buds

Also called: fire, primo, top shelf, loud, kill, chronic, dank, headies, flame, kine, kind, and a host of other regional naming trends

Effects: advanced potency and flavor profiles provide a diverse range of effects and individual experiences that amplify the consumer's connection to the cannabis plant

Everybody claims to have high-quality cannabis in stock, but how can you tell for yourself? The first thing you should know about top-shelf buds is that they will stand out in a sea of green. Besides the diverse spectrum of colors that premier genetics show, the amazing quality and complex aromas of truly dank cannabis will scream "Pick me!" The nickname "loud" is used for this exact reason, because the pungent flavors are often too much to contain and can draw attention to those who have it, especially when trying to be discreet. Truly outstanding cannabis has no price cap—it can be considered a luxury item like fine wine and, depending on the laws where you live, prices can reach extreme levels.

First-class cannabis will have a thick coat of sugary resin that contains the cannabinoids and terpenes, giving the plant its powerful effects and captivating flavors. The buds themselves are typically dense and chunky, thick from advanced CO_2 levels during the flowering cycle and other innovative growing techniques.

The harvesting, drying, and curing methods used by the grower can greatly influence the end result. Truly dank herb should be sticky from the frosting of trichomes without being moist or wet. When ground, it should break apart without becoming a pile of dust, and when burnt, it should leave behind white ash (black ash is a signal that there is excess moisture in your flowers).

Proper trimming is paramount to true connoisseurs, allowing each cola and nug to be showcased and perfectly framed. If top-shelf cannabis appears leafy, it's most often because the sugar leaves surrounding the buds are covered with trichomes too precious to discard. Seeds are extremely rare to find in the finest-quality cannabis, so if you uncover one in your stash, keep it for your own garden (providing you can legally grow in your state, of course).

How to Store Your Cannabis

LIKE WINE AND whiskey, cannabis is best when aged in a cool, dark place, and while there is no steadfast expiration date for cannabis, there are a few key elements to consider when storing your buds for any extended period.

Ideal Storage Temperatures

Mildew and other molds on cannabis and other organic matter thrive in temperatures between 77° F and 86° F, so basic precautions of keeping your cannabis in a cool, dark place will go a long way. Excessive heat can dry out the cannabinoids and terpenes that have taken months to develop. When these essential oils get too dry along with plant material, it can result in a hot, harsh smoke.

Lower temperatures also slow the process of decarboxylation of cannabinoids, the process that transfers THCA into the psychoactive THC and eventually degrades into the less desired CBN.

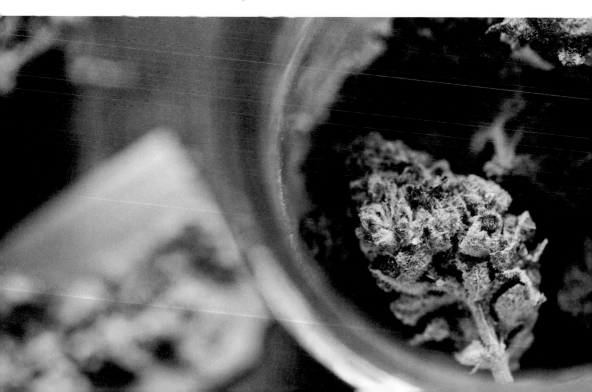

Humidity Factors

Humidity control is paramount to keeping mildew and other mold contaminants away from your cannabis. Keeping your cannabis stored in a controlled environment with the proper relative humidity (RH) ranges can be a bit of a balancing act, but the general consensus is to keep cannabis between 59 percent and 63 percent RH when stored to maintain and enhance color, consistency, aroma, and flavor. Keeping your RH below 65 percent reduces the chances for mold to occur. However, if your RH drops too low, you risk your trichomes becoming brittle and drying out the essential oils.

Light Settings

Harmful UV rays break down many organic and synthetic materials. Similar to the way your grass turns brown at the end of a long sunny summer, or how a car's paint begins to fade when it is not garaged, UV rays will degrade your cannabis over time. A study conducted at the University of London in the 1970s concluded that light was the single biggest factor in the degradation of cannabinoids. The same study concluded that cannabinoids maintain stability for up to two years when stored under the proper conditions, though they can remain effective and safe to consume for much longer as the essential oils slowly break down over time. Storing your cannabis out of direct light will also help you control the temperature.

Air Control

While cannabis needs oxygen during growing and curing, storing your cannabis in a container with just the right amount of air is crucial to keeping it fresh and true to its original form. Having too little air can greatly affect the relative humidity, especially if the buds are not completely dried before storage. Too much air, on the other hand, will speed up the degradation process as the cannabinoids and other organic matter are exposed to oxygen. There are a variety of hand and electric vacuum pump attachments available for canning jars that will help you minimize oxygen exposure.

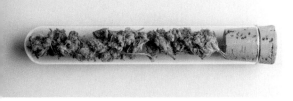

Cannabis Storage Dos

Do separate your strains to maintain their individual flavor profiles.

Do store your buds out of direct sunlight in a cool, dry place.

Do store cannabis in containers with a neutral charge, like glass jars.

Do use hygrometers or humidity control products to monitor and control RH levels.

Do vacuum seal jars and containers when storing cannabis long-term to minimize oxygen exposure.

Cannabis Storage Don'ts

Don't store your cannabis in the refrigerator; the fluctuations in humidity and temperature can actually increase the chance of mold and mildew.

Don't store your cannabis in the freezer, because freezing temperatures will cause the fragile trichomes to become brittle and break off like little icicles when handled.

Don't store buds in plastic bags or containers. Plastic often has a static charge that can attract precious trichomes. If you must use a plastic bag, only use it for short-term storage of small quantities of cannabis.

Don't store above or around electronics or appliances that give off heat. Heat rises and can negatively impact your buds. Instead, store your cannabis in a low cupboard, shelf, or in the basement of your house, much like a wine cellar.

Don't use a tobacco humidor. Most use cedar wood, which has oils that transfer and can influence the flavors of your cannabis. They also tend to employ sponges that use propylene glycol to regulate humidity and can oversaturate your cannabis.

Don't store grinders, pipes, or other paraphernalia with your cannabis. The ash and resin from burnt cannabis tends to linger and will stink up any storage container. Also, it's simply good etiquette to keep your supplies separate and clean.

Final Thoughts on Storage

Products infused with cannabis, such as edibles and other perishable creations, will have different storage guidelines. Don't store these items for long periods of time. Follow the directions on the package and store your edibles similar to ordinary food items.

Alcohol tinctures and other cannabis concentrates seem to be less susceptible to mold and other contaminants due to the reduced amount of bio matter. However, we still recommend following the basic guidelines we outlined to protect potency and minimize possible contamination.

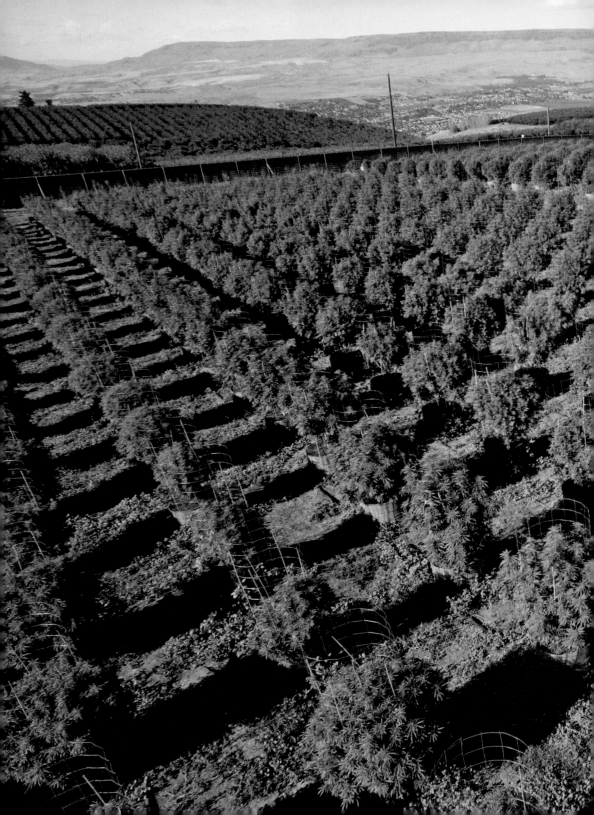

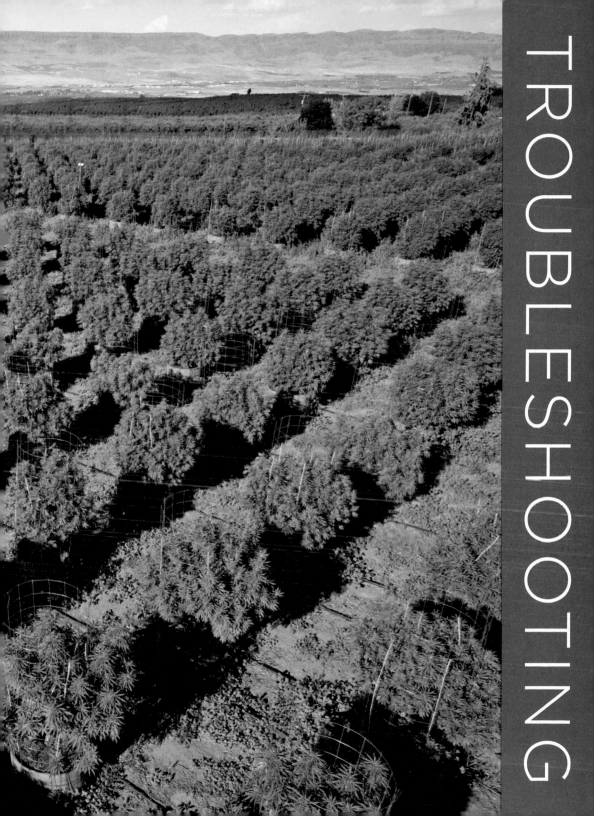

Possible Side Effects of High-THC Cannabis and How to Counteract Them

LIKE VIRTUALLY ALL medicines, cannabis can induce its own unique set of side effects. Although not everyone's experience comes with a side of adverse reactions, it's worth knowing what you may be at risk for, especially if you're a new user. Before you try cannabis that's high in THC, familiarize yourself with these common side effects so you can recognize any adverse reactions you may experience.*

* This is not a substitute for medical advice, which you should seek if needed.

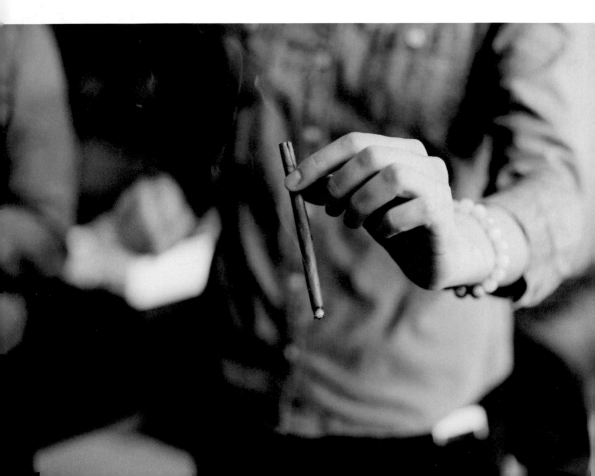

Paranoia and Anxiety

One of the worst side effects of THC is anxiety and paranoia. Though small amounts of THC are likely to induce only mild paranoia or social anxiety, edibles and large doses can cause exaggerated side effects. THC is known to relieve anxiety in smaller doses and increase it in larger applications; this is due to its biphasic effects, meaning it can have two opposite effects in high doses. Furthermore, some people are genetically predisposed to experience anxiety with cannabis as a result of brain chemistry.

Consider trying: CBD strains, which are often amazing antianxiety solutions. You may also want to only consume when you're in a comfortable, familiar place, such as at home or with trusted friends.

Dry Mouth

Better known as the dreaded "cotton-mouth," high-THC cannabis can also make your mouth drier than the Sahara Desert. Believe it or not, there are cannabinoid receptors in our saliva glands. THC mirrors a naturally occurring chemical called anandamide, which binds to these receptors to decrease saliva production. THC, with its high affinity toward these receptors, exaggerates the effect.

Consider trying: Plenty of water; remember to stay hydrated and drink lots of fluids when consuming cannabis. You may also want to start with low doses and slowly work your way up as your tolerance builds.

Dry, Red Eyes

Not only does THC cause the mouth to dry out, it can also affect the eyes. It's the classic telltale giveaway that has made eyedrops a natural companion for discreet cannabis consumers. But what causes it and are eyedrops the only cure?

It may be, in part, due to the fact that smoke can irritate the eyes, but other consumption methods can also cause dry, red eyes. THC is known to lower blood pressure and dilate blood vessels in the eyes, leading to redness. Though less likely, an allergy to cannabis can also cause red eyes.

Consider trying: Lots of water or fluids to stay hydrated. Eyedrops can be helpful if your eyes are irritated, but avoid relying on them every time, as some brands can actually cause dryness if used continually.

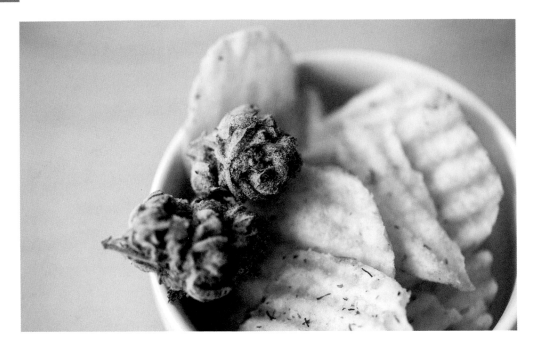

Hunger and "Munchies"

Unless you have an underactive appetite, you might consider the munchies to be an annoying side effect of THC. Because it stimulates areas of the brain associated with appetite, THC can jumpstart a fierce hunger.

Consider trying: High-CBD or high-THCV strains, which should help curb your appetite.

Sleepiness and Lethargy

This side effect is seen by some as a thera-peutic benefit as THC fights insomnia and promotes rest. However, if you're looking to stay active while using cannabis, bear in mind that some strains can induce naps, lethargy, or an early night's sleep.

Consider trying: Sativa or high-CBD strains for daytime use; try to avoid strong indica strains and save them for evening consumption (or for when you need some rest). You may also consider trying a cannabis-infused coffee or tea to help lift out the lethargy.

Impaired Memory

Although memory impairment tends to be less of a problem for new consumers, it can be an annoying affliction to many. Even short-term effects can get in the way of a productive afternoon and cognitive tasks.

Consider trying: High-CBD strains are often a wonderful alternative for anyone looking to keep their memory and cognition intact. Supplements like ginkgo biloba and B vitamins may be helpful in countering these side effects, but your best bet for maintaining cognition is dosing low and slow.

TIPS FOR AVOIDING THC'S NEGATIVE EFFECTS IN THE FIRST PLACE

If you want to be proactive before you sit down to enjoy some top-shelf cannabis or a new infused product, keep these best practices in mind to minimize the less desirable effects of THC:

- Try a strain that is high in CBD, like ACDC, Cannatonic, Harlequin, or Canna-Tsu. CBD is not psychoactive in the same way as THC, and it can help curb the side effects of THC for a more relaxed, mellow experience

- Start with a very low dose when using high-THC strains. Adverse side effects tend to set in with continued or heavy consumption, so start with just a puff or two and see how you feel. You'd be surprised how much fun you can have with minimal amounts of cannabis.

- Consider using an oil-filled vape pen if you're sensitive to smoking or edibles. These allow a great deal of dosing control with mild effects, which has made them incredibly popular choices among newcomers and older generations jumping back into cannabis.

- Start with a 5-milligram dose of edibles if you're unaccustomed to THC. From there, you can slowly and responsibly work your way up in dosage if the effects are mild.

- Drink lots of water while using cannabis. Hydration is key to avoiding many unpleasant side effects.

You may experience a number of other side effects with cannabis such as headaches, dizziness, and respiratory difficulties, although these are less common. It's always a good idea to talk to your doctor before partaking, and to communicate your cannabis consumption, particularly in case it interacts with another medication you are taking. Because its most common side effects may be mild, many patients prefer it to other medications, but familiarizing yourself with any and all risks is the best way to ensure a good experience for yourself.

What to Do If
You Get Too High

ANY CANNABIS CONSUMER can tell you there's one feeling to avoid, it's the moment when you realize, "I'm too high." Maybe the edible kicked in three hours late. Perhaps you tried to impress a group of friends by breathing in a little bit too deeply. You might have just tried concentrates for the first time and were caught off-guard by their potency. Or maybe you just have a low tolerance to cannabis. There are a thousand ways it can happen, but once it does, the resulting experience can be uncomfortable at best and enough to turn off even the most seasoned cannabis lover.

Fear not! Most of us have experienced the unpleasantness that can come with overwhelming cannabis effects. Thankfully, there are ways to help come back down when you feel too high, overwhelmed, uncomfortable, or ill from excessive cannabis consumption.

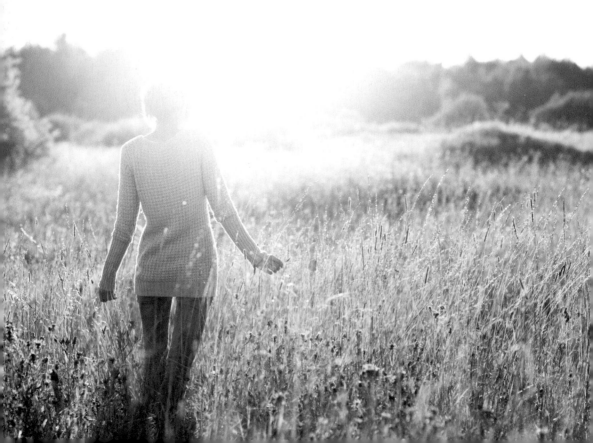

1. Don't Panic

Let us start with the infinite wisdom of *The Hitchhiker's Guide to the Galaxy*:

> **Don't panic. You are fine
> and everything is okay.**

Most symptoms of "greening out" (consuming too much cannabis) will dissipate within minutes to hours, with no lasting effects beyond a little grogginess. Give it some time and these feelings will eventually past, trust us.

2. Know Your Limits Before Consuming

If you can, try to prepare for your cannabis session according to your tolerance level. Consume with friends you know and are comfortable with, and don't feel pressured to consume more than you can handle. It's all well and good to make new friends, but being surrounded by strangers when you feel ill is unpleasant at best and anxiety-inducing at worst.

Take it slow, especially when consuming edibles. If you're trying edibles for the first time, start out with a standard dose of 10 milligrams (or even 5 milligrams if you really want to ease into the experience) and wait at least an hour, if not two, before increasing your edibles dosage. The same goes for inhalation methods—if you're used to occasionally taking one hit off your

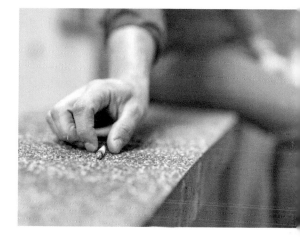

personal vaporizer, don't abruptly upgrade to sitting in a smoking circle puffing and passing for an hour without first slowly increasing your tolerance.

3. Hydrate

Water, water, water—don't forget to hydrate! Whether you prefer water or juice, make sure you have a nice, cold beverage on hand (preferably caffeine-free). This will help you combat dry mouth and allow you to focus on a simple and familiar act: sipping and swallowing.

"Hydrate," by the way, does not mean "knock back a few alcoholic beverages." If you're feeling the effects of your strain a little too aggressively, stay away from alcohol as it can significantly increase THC blood concentrations and make effects feel more intense.

4. Keep Some Black Pepper on Hand

If you find yourself combating paranoia and anxiety, a simple household ingredient found in kitchens and restaurants everywhere can come to your rescue: black pepper. According to a scientific review published by Ethan Russo in the *British Journal of Pharmacology*, cannabis and pepper have very similar chemical traits; pepper has a "phytocannabinoid-terpenoid effect," which is known to help with pain, depression, addiction, and anxiety. Combining the terpenoids (such as beta-caryophyllene) in pepper with the tetrahydrocannabinol in cannabis has a synergistic chemical reaction on the cannabinoid receptors in the brain.

In layman's terms, they both bind to the same receptors in the brain and, when combined, have a therapeutic, calming effect.

Many swear by the black pepper trick, so if too much cannabis has you on the verge of freaking out, just sniff or chew on a few black peppercorns for almost instantaneous relief.

5. Keep Calm, Rest, and Nap

Find a calm, quiet place where you can rest and breathe deeply. Remember, the intense discomfort you're feeling will pass. Take deep full breaths in through your nose and out through your mouth. Focus on the sound of your breath and just rest a while.

Sometimes sleeping it off can be the best alternative for stopping a strong high, but it's not always easy to turn your brain off. Once you've found a quiet area, lie down and let yourself relax. If drowsiness and sleep are quick to occur, take a little nap to rejuvenate yourself. Should you be unable to fall asleep, just get comfortable until you feel strong enough to spring back up.

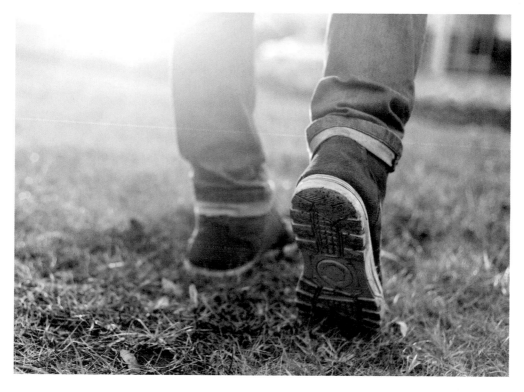

6. Try Going for a Walk

If you can't turn your brain off, sometimes a change of scenery and some fresh air to get your blood pumping will help invigorate you. Just remember to stay close to your immediate surroundings— don't wander off and get lost while you're feeling sick, anxious, or paranoid! Refrain from taking a walk if you're too woozy or light-headed to stand.

7. Take a Shower or Bath

While it's not always feasible if you're out and about or at a friend's house, if you're at home, try taking a nice shower or bath as a pleasant way to help you relax. As always, it's best to have someone else there if you don't feel well.

8. Distract Yourself

All of the activities that seem so entertaining and fun while high are also a great way to distract yourself while you try to come back down to earth. Some suggestions include:

- Watch a funny cartoon

- Listen to your favorite album

- Play a fun video game

- Talk to your friends (who are hopefully right by your side, reassuring you)

- Snuggle with your significant other

- Try coloring as a calming activity

- Eat something delicious

Whatever distractions you prefer, make sure it's a familiar activity that gives you warm, fuzzy emotions. Your brain will hopefully zone in on the positive feelings and give you a gentle reminder that you are safe and just fine.

9. Try a High-CBD Strain or Product

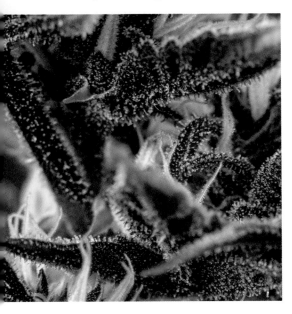

CBD is an excellent anxiety-fighting compound, and for many people it can be used to counteract too much THC. It has been found to enhance THC's painkilling properties while diminishing the paranoia it can cause. If you have a high-CBD strain that's low in THC, try taking a few puffs of it to balance out the anxiety or paranoia you're experiencing from another strain.

Of course, you can always seek medical attention and tell a doctor or nurse that you are having a cannabis-induced anxiety attack. From a medical perspective, physicians have your best interest in mind and want to do all they can to make sure you're okay, even if it's helping you come down when you're too stoned.

Can You Overdose from Cannabis?

THE NUMBER OF people who have died due to cannabis overdose, in all of recorded history, is twenty. But keep in mind that while cannabis itself cannot kill the human body, it is very possible to "overdose" on cannabis in the sense of overconsumption. Most experienced cannabis consumers have, at one point or another, gotten to a place they didn't want to be. Perhaps you didn't check the dosage on that edible and now you're regretting it. You're uncomfortable or sick. You may be feeling downright miserable. Your discomfort, as wretched as it may be, will pass. (See the previous section, What to Do If You Get Too High.)

Why is that, exactly?

It's possible to die from opioid overdose or alcohol poisoning. But cannabis

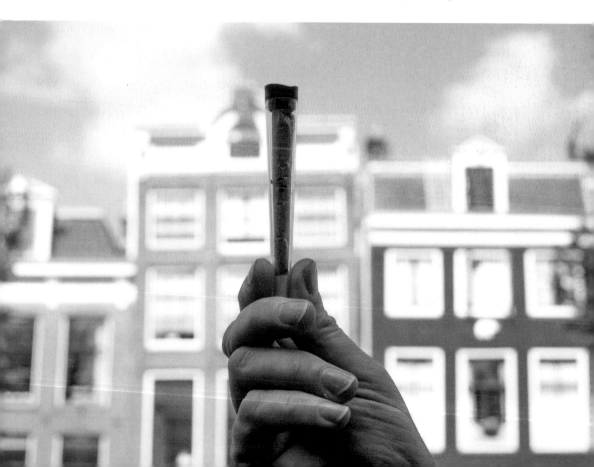

acts on the body and mind in a way that's very different from opioids or alcohol.

We're all familiar with the tragic phrase "died of an overdose," but when opioids like fentanyl, OxyContin, or heroin are the cause, there's a specific mechanism that leads to death. As Oxford University anesthesiology professor K. T. S. Pattinson has observed, "In drug addicts, respiratory depression is the major cause of death." In other words, during an opioid overdose the victim falls unconscious and the body forgets to breathe.

What scientists call "the fundamental drive to respiration"—i.e., what tells the body to breathe—originates low in the brain stem, in an area known as the pre-Bötzinger complex. Opioids don't just suppress pain and increase feelings of pleasure; they also depress the pre-Bötzinger complex, which causes breathing to become slow and irregular. In an overdose, breathing shuts down completely and death occurs due to lack of oxygen. In some cases, an opioid overdose can also depress the brain's mechanism that regulates the heart and blood circulation, leading to a drop in blood pressure and heart failure.

Alcohol poisoning can become lethal when the alcohol overwhelms the liver's ability to clear it, and the blood alcohol anesthetizes the brain systems that regulate breathing and blood pressure. They shut down, which leads to death.

Why doesn't cannabis have the same effect? Because cannabinoids act on specific receptors that are not concentrated in the brain stem, where breathing and heart rate are controlled.

Cannabinoid receptors are most highly concentrated in the basal ganglia, the hippocampus, and cerebellum, which control cognition and movement. Those same receptors appear in scant numbers in brain-stem areas like the pre-Bötzinger complex.

In a 1990 study of cannabinoid receptors, researchers with the National Institutes of Health (NIH) reported that "sparse densities [of cannabinoid receptors] in lower brain stem areas controlling cardiovascular and respiratory functions may explain why high doses of THC are not lethal."

In summary, opioid and alcohol overdose can shut down the body's breathing and blood circulatory systems, located in the lower brain stem. Cannabis does not have the ability to affect those lower brain stem systems in the same way. While it's very possible to overdo your cannabis intake, it's not possible to die from a cannabis overdose.

How Long Does THC Stay in Your System?

A COMMON QUESTION for cannabis consumers, especially those who are concerned about workplace drug testing, is how long THC lingers in the body. Before we dive into a suitable answer, it's important to keep in mind two key caveats:

1. There are many different kinds of drug tests available, which have varying levels of sensitivity and time periods to detect cannabis in your system.

2. Wide-ranging patterns of usage as well as a unique biology for each individual make the calculation of a concrete detection window (the number of days after ceasing usage that a drug test will continue to be positive) even more complex.

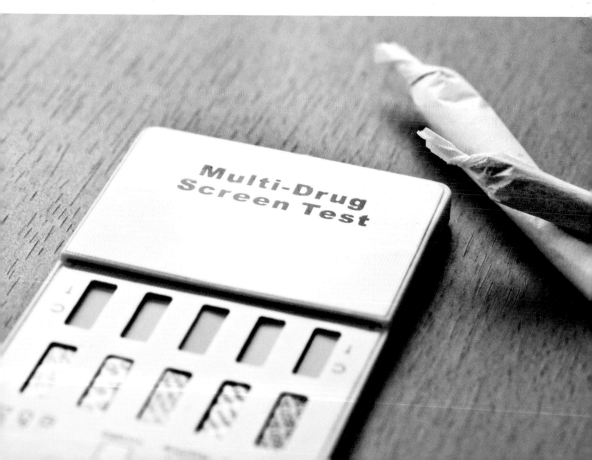

How Do Drug Tests Work?

About forty to fifty million drug tests are conducted by employers each year, which analyze biological material including urine, hair, blood, saliva, breath, sweat, and even fingernails. When cannabis is consumed, THC levels temporarily rise in the body, which are detectable by blood tests from several hours up to a day after a single usage. Although these levels drop significantly after a few days, there are still other means of determining recent usage.

THC, CBD, and their metabolic by-products (called metabolites) are lipid-soluble and accumulate in fat reserves throughout the body. These molecules are then slowly released over time, resulting in a considerably longer time period for the body to purge itself of marijuana traces compared to other recreational drugs, especially for chronic users.

> Hair tests tend to have the longest detection window, capable of registering the levels of a nonpsychoactive THC metabolite called 11-nor-delta9-caboxy-THC (THC-COOH) up to ninety days after cessation.

While each drug test has its advantages, urine tests tend to be the test of choice for most private employers and are the sole test recommended by the Substance Abuse and Mental Health Services Administration (SAMHSA), a branch of the U.S. Department of Health and Human Services that sets standards for drug testing of government employees. Urine screens do not directly measure the amount of THC present, but rather the levels of the metabolite THC-COOH.

Once a specific test is selected, the experimenter must then choose its sensitivity, or the cutoff concentration of THC-COOH above which a test is considered positive. The most common cutoff for most urine tests is 50 nanograms per milliliter (ng/ml), but cutoffs can be as low as 15 ng/ml and as high as 100 ng/ml, each of which result in widely different detection windows.

Despite the fact that SAMHSA sets standards that regulate these urine tests, the vast variability in cannabis use as well as individual differences in biology and genetics make it difficult to develop specific time windows for detection.

How Long Does Cannabis Stay in Your System?

Each of us has a unique metabolism that processes cannabis at a different rate, further complicating the picture. Even among people of the same gender and age, individual lifestyle choices such as levels of exercise and eating habits may also affect the amount of time required to pass a drug test (those with higher levels of fat content store cannabinoids more readily than leaner folks).

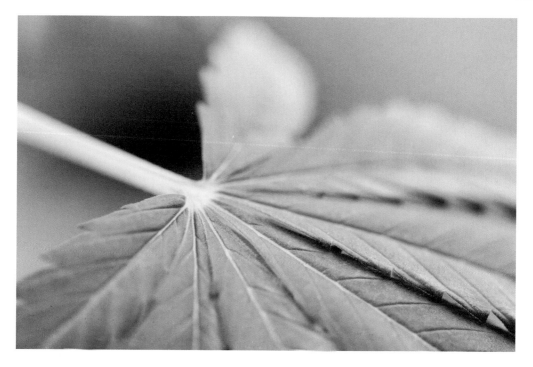

While detection times in excess of thirty days do occur for some, they are largely an exception. For example, a 1989 study of chronic users showed a maximum detection window of twenty-five days at a sensitivity of 20 ng/ml. Yet only one subject tested positive after fourteen days, and it took an average of just 9.8 days before cannabinoid levels were no longer detectible. And while a 1984 study testing chronic users at a cutoff of 50 ng/ml showed a maximum of forty days to get clean, eight out of the ten subjects needed only thirteen days to show their first negative.

These findings are general recommendations, not hard facts; actual detection windows will vary based on a number of factors outlined in this chapter.

Chronic* users at the standard 50 ng/ml cutoff: unlikely detection for longer than 10 days after last smoking session

Chronic users at 20 ng/ml: unlikely detection for longer than 21 days after last smoking session

First-time/occasional* users at the standard 50 ng/ml cutoff: unlikely detection for longer than 3 to 4 days after last smoking session

First time/occasional users at 20 ng/ml: unlikely detection for longer than 7 days after last smoking session

*"Occasional" and "chronic" each represent opposite sides of the usage spectrum, with most users likely falling somewhere in the middle.

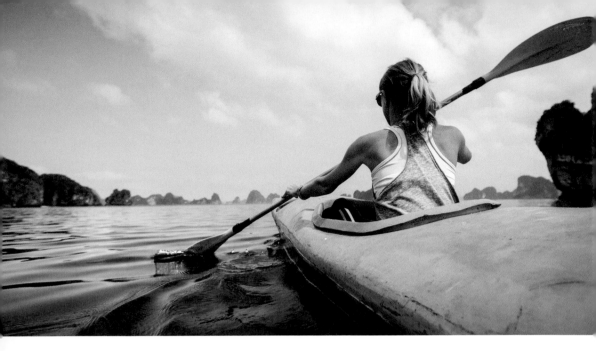

Factors That May Impact Drug Test Results

There are instances where individuals fluctuate between positive and negative tests over a period of time. A couple of factors may contribute to a range of variability in positive THC tests:

- Dehydration—if a person becomes dehydrated, it concentrates the urine, which can increase the chance of a positive test

- Exercise—working out breaks down fat cells and releases THC, which can spike levels detected in a drug test

How Long Does CBD Stay in Your System, and Will it Show Up on a Drug Test?

Because standard urine testing only analyzes metabolites of THC, those who consume CBD or CBD hemp oil have very little risk of testing positive. Hemp oils contain very small amounts of THC. If you use an extraordinarily large amount of cannabinoid-rich oil products (greater than 1,000 to 2,000 milligrams each day), you might show a positive test on the initial urine screen, which is susceptible to cross-contamination from other cannabinoids. However, this initial "false positive" would not hold up to the more rigorous second round of confirmatory testing, which specifically measures THC-COOH.

Can You "Cheat" a Cannabis Drug Test?

Is there anything you can do to prevent a positive test or speed up the detoxification process?

Although abstinence is an obvious initial answer, it may even be dangerous to hang out with friends who are smoking. In a 2015 study, a small group of participants were exposed to secondhand smoke in both ventilated and unventilated rooms. Some participants who sat in the unventilated room tested positive for THC-COOH, with concentrations in urine exceeding 57 ng/ml. While it's not a given that being exposed to secondhand cannabis smoke will result in a positive drug test, it is possible, so if you're subject to drug testing and are surrounded by a group of people smoking cannabis in a confined space, you should leave.

Will Eating Hemp Foods Result in a Positive Drug Test for THC?

Regular consumption or use of commercially made hemp foods (such as seeds, cooking oil, cereals, milk, granola) or hemp products (lotions, shampoos, lip balms, et cetera) will not show a positive result for THC on a drug test. Hemp-based foods and hemp body products commercially produced and sold in the United States are not legally allowed to contain THC. If a laboratory-tested hemp product did happen to contain trace amounts of this compound, it would be in such small quantities that it would likely require exorbitant amounts of ingestion or use for it to even remotely begin to show up in the smallest amount on a drug test. With that said, consuming noncommercially produced hemp foods, hemp-based oils, or using homemade hemp-based products may risk a positive test result. Nonfederally regulated foods and products, like those purchased from a dispensary, farmer's market, or even products bought online, do not necessarily follow any sort of federal food safety guidelines or Food and Drug Administration regulations. When purchasing these types of hemp products, make sure you use caution and ask questions about how they were made and whether they were tested before being packaged.

How to Get Rid of THC in Your System

For those who are able to quit, one common technique is to flush out your system by drinking a lot of water. This can be a good approach, as dehydration will increase the concentration of your urine and could increase your chances for a positive result. If your urine is diluted too much, however, it will automatically invalidate the results and you will have to repeat the test, so hydrate carefully.

A potentially more effective tactic for speeding up the detoxification process

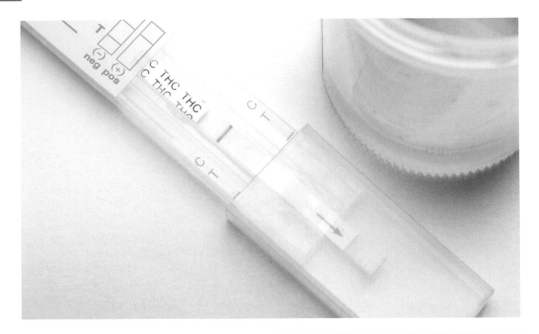

might be cutting back on the burgers and hitting the gym. People with more fat will have more tissue for cannabinoid storage, so they might experience a slightly longer window of detection. Fasting will burn fat, which will in turn release more cannabinoids.

Make sure to give your body enough time to clear out these stored cannabinoids, as exercise or fasting will likely result in a transient spike in measurable THC metabolites as they exit the body.

If you know you have an upcoming drug test, not all hope is lost. Given the current detection windows for standard cannabis tests, it's likely you will be able to pass a urine test as long as you are not an extremely heavy user and are given sufficient advance notice.

Many who are facing a drug test but are unwilling to fully give up cannabis turn to synthetic cannabinoids in the hopes of cheating traditional tests. These alternatives, commonly referred to as "K2" or "spice," are unpredictable, showing side effects ranging from nausea to seizures that have caused a spike in overdoses and even deaths. And many private companies now include tests for synthetic cannabinoids in their repertoire, making this approach both dangerous and futile. Bottom line: Stay far, far away from synthetic cannabis. It's dangerous.

Others who continue to smoke may attempt to tamper with their urine, adding chemicals such as pyridinium chlorochromate or peroxidase that eliminate THC-COOH in the sample. Most testing agencies, however, will screen for these compounds, and being caught is often just as bad, if not worse, than a positive test.

What Is a "Tolerance Break"?

REGULAR CANNABIS CONSUMERS have been known to experience fluctuations in their tolerance to marijuana over time. Despite rotating strains or trying new consumption methods, some consumers report that the expected effects from cannabis seem to dissipate or feel muted after repeated use. To combat these diminishing effects, some consumers opt to take "tolerance breaks" in order to refresh how their bodies and minds react to cannabis.

A tolerance break, sometimes called a t-break, is just that: a short-term break from cannabis to clear one's head and body of cannabinoids, notably THC. But does it work? Past research has indicated that regular cannabis consumers do indeed build up a tolerance to the drug.

A study by Dr. Miles Herkenham of the National Institute of Mental Health on the cannabinoid receptor system and its tolerance to cannabis came to the following conclusion:

> The effect . . . is time- and dose-dependent, and is reversible, and thus appears to be cannabinoid-receptor mediated . . . The result [of the study] has implications for the consequences of chronic high levels of drug use in humans, suggesting diminishing effects with greater levels of consumption.

While it's possible to become highly tolerant of cannabis and its myriad effects, the buildup can be reversed by taking a break from the drug. Some consumers

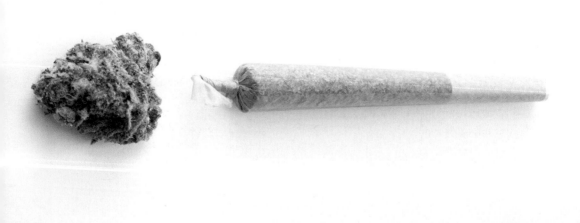

benefit from reducing their rate of consumption, while others choose to abstain completely for a set duration so that the more noticeable, psychoactive effects of cannabis can return at fuller potency.

A tolerance break can also consist of changing a consumer's regular routine, which can influence the effectiveness of cannabis and the way it interacts with the mind and body. For example, skipping consumption in the morning may encourage the onset of stronger effects during evening consumption. Ultimately, the length and severity of a tolerance break depends on the individual and their consumption patterns.

How Long Should a Cannabis Tolerance Break Last?

Since cannabis is a highly individualistic experience, a tolerance break can take on many forms depending on one's consumption pattern. Generally speaking, a few days without cannabis should be enough to begin to notice the return of more profound effects, while abstaining for a week or two is recommended to help get a consumer over the hump and shake up his or her usual routine. Once the mind has acclimated to its new clear-headed groove and the body has adjusted accordingly, it's a good sign that the t-break has taken hold.

For those looking to flush their body completely, try pushing past the two-week mark, as THC and other compounds can remain in one's system for more than thirty days.

What Should Consumers Expect on a Cannabis Tolerance Break?

During a tolerance break, try staying active and hydrating often. Working out at the gym, playing sports, hiking, and engaging in other physical activities will help make pressing the "reset" button more impactful, as will eating right and focusing on good nutrition habits. Try going for a run, cooking a healthy meal, or taking on a hobby that will offer some positive reward or self-satisfaction.

Consumers who opt to take a tolerance break should remember that when they make their return to the plant, it's important to scale back the quantity that's typically consumed. The longer the break taken, the further down the ladder one should start; otherwise, there's a risk of feeling overwhelmed by the potency and effects that once seemed muted or manageable.

Acknowledgments

This book was put together with the help of the entire Leafly team. From sales and marketing to operations, product and engineering, what makes Leafly unique is our group's genuine desire to share information and tell great stories. Ideas come to us from partners in the industry, from our colleagues at our parent and sister companies, and from our readers across the world. Without their perspectives, this book would not be possible.

Huge thanks to the Leafly News group, all of whom put enormous effort into making this book what it is. Bruce Barcott, Ben Adlin, Gage Peake, Dave Schmader, Hannah Meadows, Lisa Rough, David Karalis, Ian Chant, Jeremiah Wilhelm, and Will Hyde; your work in making cannabis an accessible topic is critical and exceptional. Special thanks to Rebecca Kelley, Brett Konen, and Bailey Rahn, for sinking nights and weekends into the writing and editing of this manuscript. And to Julia Sumpter, for your tireless and incomparable photography and image sourcing.

Sean Desmond, who brought this idea to Leafly in 2016 and drove its mission and vision, and Rachel Kambury, who saw the book through production, are two of the best partners you could ever ask for in publishing. Thank you both for your commitment to this ambitious project.

—*Sam Martin, Editor-in Chief*

Works Consulted

Borges et al., "Understanding the Molecular Aspects of Tetrahydrocannabinol and Cannabidiol as Antioxidants." *Molecules.* 2013.

Gates et al., "Cannabis smoking and respiratory health: consideration of the literature." *Respirology.* 2014.

Herkenham et al., "Cannabinoid receptor localization in brain." *Proceedings of the National Academy of Sciences.* 1990.

Lee & Hancox, "Effects of smoking cannabis on lung function." *Expert Review of Respiratory Medicine.* 2011.

Naeher et al., "Woodsmoke health effects: a review." *Inhalation Toxicology.* 2007.

Nagarkatti et al., "Cannabinoids as Novel Anti-inflammatory Drugs." *Future Medicinal Chemistry.* 2009.

Ständer et al., "Distribution of Cannabinoid Receptor 1 (CB1) and 2 (CB2) on Sensory Nerve Fibers and Adnexal Structures in Human Skin." *Journal of Dermatological Science.* 2005.

Tashkin, "Effects of marijuana smoking on the lung." *Annals of the American Thoracic Society.* 2013.

Van der Kooy et al., "Cannabis Smoke Condensate I: The Effect of Different Preparation Methods on Tetrahydrocannabinol Levels." *Inhalation Toxicology.* 2008.

Wang et al., "One Minute of Marijuana Secondhand Smoke Exposure Substantially Impairs Vascular Endothelial Function." *Journal of the American Heart Association.* 2016.

Wester et al., "Benzene Levels in Ambient Air and Breath of Smokers and Nonsmokers in Urban and Pristine Environments." *Journal of Toxicology Environmental Health.* 1986.

Wilkinson et al., "Cannabinoids Inhibit Human Keratinocyte Proliferation through a Non-CB1/CB2 Mechanism and Have a Potential Therapeutic Value in the Treatment of Psoriasis." *Journal of Dermatological Science.* 2007.

Helpful Resources

Americans for Safe Access: The ASA aims to provide safe and legal access to cannabis for therapeutic use and research. They are a hub for medical information, legal information, and more. Find them at safeaccessnow.org.

Drug Policy Alliance: The DPA is one of the nation's leading organizations in promoting drug policy reform. They provide information and facts about science and health at drugpolicy.org.

Harm Reduction Therapy Center: This center is a certified drug and alcohol treatment program staffed by mental health professionals. Find them at harmreductiontherapy.org

Illustration Credits

1: Getty/iStock, Simon Skafar; 2: Getty/iStock, Kosamtu; 3: Getty/iStock, SEASTOCK; 4: Getty/iStock, Boris Vasilenko; 5: Getty/iStock, Jens Gade; 6: Getty/iStock, TH Collins Photography; 7: Leafly, Julia Sumpter; 8: Getty/iStock, Natan Bolckmans; 9: Leafly, Julia Sumpter; 10: Getty/iStock, irina88w; 11: Leafly, Adrienne Allen; 12: Leafly; 13: Leafly, Adrienne Allen; 14: Getty/iStock, Franck Reporter; 15: Leafly, Adrienne Allen; 16: Getty/iStock, portishead1; 17: Leafly/Adrienne Allen; 18: Getty/iStock, razerbird; 19: Getty/iStock, eskymaks; 20: Getty/iStock, pkripper503; 21: Leafly/Adrienne Allen; 22: Leafly/Adrienne Allen; 23: Getty/iStock, Wonderland Productions; 24: Leafly/Adrienne Allen; 25: Leafly/Adrienne Allen; 26: Getty/iStock, dkhoriaty; 27: Getty/iStock, ksushachmeister; 28: Getty/iStock, contrastaddict; 29: Getty/iStock, Helios8; 30: Leafly/Adrienne Allen; 31: Leafly/Adrienne Allen; 32: Getty/iStock, Pe3check; 33: Getty/iStock, gabe9000c; 34: Leafly/Adrienne Allen; 35: Getty/iStock, Don Bayley; 36: Getty/iStock, Pekic; 37: Getty/iStock, InnerVisionPRO; 38: Getty/iStock, belterz; 39: Leafly/Adrienne Allen; 40: Leafly; 41: Getty/iStock, monkeybusinessimages; 42: Leafly/Adrienne Allen; 43: Leafly/Julia Sumpter; 44: Getty/iStock, KIVILCIM PINAR; 45: Leafly/Julia Sumpter; 46: Getty/iStock, Sergey Moskvitin; 47: Getty/iStock, andykatz; 48: Getty/iStock, JANIFEST; 49: Leafly/Julia Sumpter; 50: Getty/iStock, Juanmonino; 51: Getty/iStock, temmuz can arsiray; 52: Getty/iStock, Carlos Restrepo; 53: Getty/iStock, Roxana Gonzalez; 54: Getty/iStock, pkripper503; 55: Leafly/Julia Sumpter; 56: Getty/iStock, jacoblund; 57: Getty/iStock, TommL; 58: Getty/iStock, morrowlight; 59: Getty/iStock, Gleti; 60: Getty/iStock, annebaek; 61: Getty/iStock; 62: Getty/iStock, YinYang; 63: Getty/iStock, alika1712; 64: Getty/iStock, Synergee; 65: Leafly/Adrienne Allen; 66: Getty/Istock, David Kerkoff; 67: Getty/iStock, momcilog; 68: Getty/iStock, VeselovaElena; 69: Getty/iStock, rez-art; 70: Getty/iStock, tyncho; 71: Getty/iStock, YelenaYemchuk; 72: Getty/iStock, Nicolas McComber; 73: Getty/iStock, Ridofranz; 74: Flickr Creative Commons/Andres Rodriguez; 75: Leafly/Julia Sumpter; 76: Leafly/Julia Sumpter; 77: Leafly/Julia Sumpter; 78: Leafly/Julia Sumpter; 79: Leafly/Julia Sumpter; 80: Leafly/Julia Sumpter; 81: Leafly/Julia Sumpter; 82: Getty/iStock, seastock; 83: Getty/iStock, Alain Studio; 84: Getty/iStock, RyanJLane; 85: Getty/iStock, petekarici; 86: Getty/iStock, ksushachmeister; 87: Getty/iStock, kmatija; 88: Getty/iStock, Roxana Gonzalez; 89: Getty/iStock, martin-dm; 90: Getty/iStock, pixdeluxe; 91: Getty/iStock, Juanmonino; 92: Getty/iStock, MmeEmil; 93: Getty/iStock, Seth Anderson; 94: Getty/iStock, ksushachmeister; 95: Getty/iStock, beusbeus; 96: Leafly/Adrienne Allen; 97: Leafly/Julia Sumpter; 98: Getty/iStock, petrunjela; 99: Getty/iStock, piola666; 100: Getty/iStock, InnerVisionPRO; 101: Getty/iStock, Vladdeep; 102: Getty/iStock, Alain Studio; 103: Getty/iStock, levers2007; 104: Getty/iStock, RapidEye; 105: Getty/iStock, rrenis2000; 106: Getty/iStock, mihtiander; 107: Getty/iStock, SageElyse; 108: Leafly/Adrienne Allen; 109: Leafly/Julia Sumpter; 110: Leafly/Julia Sumpter; 111: Leafly/Julia Sumpter; 112: Leafly/Julia Sumpter; 113: Leafly/Julia Sumpter

Index

MISSION STATEMENT

Twelve strives to publish singular books, by authors who have unique perspectives and compelling authority. Books that explain our culture; that illuminate, inspire, provoke, and entertain. Our mission is to provide a consummate publishing experience for our authors, one truly devoted to thoughtful partnership and cutting-edge promotional sophistication that reaches as many readers as possible. For readers, we aim to spark that rare reading experience—one that opens doors, transports, and possibly changes their outlook on our ever-changing world.